HOW SHIFT WORK BREAKS YOUR BIOLOGY

THE
SHIFT WORKERS
PARADOX

R.E. HENGSTERMAN, RN

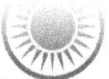

CIRCADIAN
PRESS

"You must never confuse faith that you will prevail in the end—which you can never afford to lose—with the discipline to confront the most brutal facts of your current reality."

—ADMIRAL JAMES STOCKDALE

Contents

Part 1: Foundational Support - Stability in an Unstable System

Part 2: Targeted Support - Precision in the Midst of Chaos

Part 3: Precision That Requires Partnership

Part 4: Where the Tradeoffs Live

Author's Note

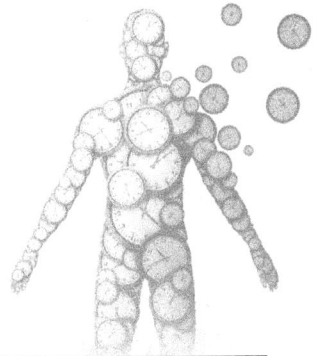

I spent over thirty years as a registered nurse—more than a decade on the night shift. One truth became painfully clear: night shift is an evolutionary mismatch that cuts deep. Modernity sharpens the blade—progress on one edge, collapse on the other.

Beyond the bedside, I built a parallel career in writing, authoring hundreds of works, from short stories in literary fiction to courses in nursing education.

At my core, I am both nurse and writer.

I know the disorienting hum of a hospital at 3 a.m., and the white-knuckled drive home as the sun rises, fighting off relentless sleep, one blink from collapse. I've suffered the demands of this life: the quiet erosion of health, the strain it places on families, the slow unraveling of the body's most vital rhythms. And I've watched it wear down my colleagues just the same.

That's what makes this book personal. If just one person feels more prepared, more informed, more in control, that alone is enough.

What follows isn't meant to be earth-shattering—it's meant to remind you of what has always been true. Across millennia, humans have relied on storytelling to bind us together, empathy kept alive around campfires.

Today, it burns under fluorescence: in nursing stations, breakrooms, factory floors, and warehouses.

This is my campfire story, rooted in time-tested wisdom. Sleep. Food. Light. Movement.

What I'm asking of you, and what I've asked of myself, is simple: place yourself under observation. Then ask, what does it feel like to be at your best?

Calm. Competent. Connected.

Let's see if, together, we can shift the behaviors that may be shifting you. And most of all, trust in the power of you.

Your physiology is built for survival. It lets you exhale, trusting the next breath will follow. Trust that next breath as you begin to trust yourself. But trust alone is not enough in a system that grinds us down.

On the surface, the shift workers of our 24/7 society—nurses, medics, police officers, factory workers—appear intact. They show up. They push through. They get the job done.

The truth is simple: the cost of working against the clock is insidious and cumulative. Yet science offers no absolutes, reminding us to stay adaptive, curious, and ready to ask better questions.

Physiological truths don't live at the extremes. They live in the middle, where nuance and evidence intersect.

The same is true for shift workers: suspended between survival and optimal health. That is *The Shift Worker's Paradox*—for those who trade sunlight for survival, yet still choose to fight for resilience, vitality, and life itself.

The Hard Truth

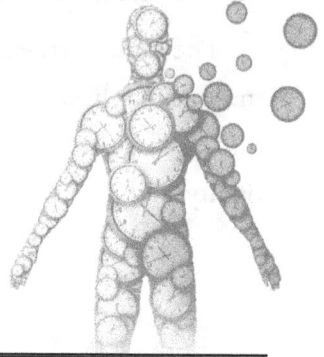

For a shift worker, the most dangerous part of the job isn't always in the operating room or on the factory floor.

It's the drive home.

It's the final stretch, the quiet miles when adrenaline slips away, and exhaustion settles in. Behind the wheel, biology becomes the enemy. And even a single death on this road is one too many.

November 5, 2013—Lauren Ryder, WNEP News

WEST CHILLISQUAQUE TOWNSHIP, PA — A two-vehicle crash on Tuesday morning in Northumberland County claimed the life of a 22-year-old woman. According to police, the crash occurred around 8:30 a.m. on Route 45 near Milton when Megan Dilick, of Millville, lost control of her car, crossed the center line, and collided head-on with a minivan.

The driver of the minivan, a critical care doctor at Geisinger, attempted to save Dilick at the scene. Despite his efforts, police confirmed that Dilick later died at the hospital.[1]

Authorities stated that Dilick was wearing a seat belt and there is no current indication of speeding...

Megan Dilick was a registered nurse and had just completed an overnight shift. She was driving home at the time of the crash. Though not attributed to fatigue, the circumstances of this crash echo the body of evidence linking roadway fatalities to cognitive impairment for shift workers, whether due to sleep loss, stress, or environmental hazards. There is no guarantee she fell asleep at the wheel; what is certain is that she had just come off a twelve-hour overnight shift, a schedule that leaves little margin for error when biology collides with the demands of the road.

Twelve years later, a similar tragedy unfolds, an echo down a different highway.

March 25, 2025 – Fox 5 Atlanta News

FORSYTH COUNTY, Ga. — Police arrested a 24-year-old nurse in connection with a crash that killed a 72-year-old earlier this month.[2]

At 8:17 a.m. on March 6, Forsyth County deputies responded to a two-vehicle crash... Forsyth County officials said a blue 2017 Volkswagen Passat had crashed into a white 2005 Chevrolet Tahoe...

Deputies spoke with the driver of the Volkswagen, later identified as 24-year-old Kayla Proctor. She told deputies she was a nurse at Northside Forsyth Hospital and was driving home from working the night shift. "Her shift was twelve and a half hours long, and this was her third night shift in a row," the report said.

Proctor told authorities she fell asleep while driving... Just before 11 a.m., medical staff pronounced [the other driver] dead.

The sheriff's office arrested Proctor and charged her with homicide by vehicle in the second degree.

Two nurses, two tragedies, one devastating link: the drive home. These are snapshots of a hidden epidemic, one where drowsy driving is a factor in one of every five fatal crashes on our roads.[3] For the shift worker, this risk is amplified, a collision between human biology and the demands of a 24/7 world. Fatigue becomes an unseen passenger, as dangerous as any mechanical failure.

And now, a terrifying precedent is being set. In the case of Kayla Proctor, we are witnessing a dangerous shift, from tragedy to criminalization. A healthcare worker, exhausted by a system that demands performance at the expense of biology, is now being held personally responsible for the physiological consequences of that exhaustion.

This ignores a fundamental truth: fatigue is not a moral failing. It is not weakness. It is not a lack of effort. Fatigue is biology. It is the unavoidable cost of sustained sleep deprivation, a condition now being treated not as a public health failure, but as a criminal offense.

And for those who still need proof, who believe drowsy driving is rare or exaggerated, science has caught up.

In a landmark study that was both elegantly simple and terrifyingly real, researchers put sixteen actual night-shift workers behind the wheel of a real car on a closed driving track, each one fresh off an eight-hour-plus shift. EEG monitors tracked brain activity. Eye-tracking cameras followed every blink. The workers were asked to drive for two hours. Then, each participant repeated the same drive—this time, after a full night of restorative sleep.

The results were a warning call. [4]

These stories are not included to sensationalize, nor to provoke pity or stir outrage for effect. They are included because they reflect the daily reality of shift workers. The names and dates may change, but the pattern does not.

These are not flukes.

They are systemic—predictable, preventable, and largely ignored.

What happens when biology is pushed past its limits? When institutional systems demand performance without pause? When rest becomes a liability, and sleep is treated as optional? To ignore these outcomes would be the greatest disservice, to the individuals lost, the professionals criminalized, and the millions still at risk.

Tragedy is a signal, a flare in the dark, warning of what we've refused to face. If we do not confront these realities directly—without euphemism, without shame—we cannot begin to change them.

And nowhere is that reality starker than in the moments after the shift ends. In controlled studies, more than one-third of drivers required an emergency braking intervention to prevent a crash.[4] Nearly half the tests, 47 percent, were stopped early because the driver dangerously lost control of the vehicle. Lane departures more than doubled.[4] By contrast, after a full night of sleep, there were zero such incidents.[4] The signs of impairment appeared with alarming speed. While the most critical failures happened after 45 minutes, the first indicators—slower reaction times, inconsistent steering, and the tell-tale slow eye movements of microsleep—emerged within just fifteen minutes.[4] This is the hard truth: for a shift worker, the danger begins almost the moment they leave the parking lot.

These findings confirm the central premise of this book: sleep is a non-negotiable biological necessity. When a system denies its workers this fundamental need, it does more than harm their personal health; it destabilizes the very fabric of public safety.

The responsibility for this cannot rest solely on the shoulders of the individual shift worker—forced to endure, adapt, and sacrifice while the system remains dangerously unchanged. Fatigue is not a personal failure. It is a physiological certainty. And yet, we continue to place the burden of survival on those who are least supported and most biologically at risk.

Protecting those who protect us requires more than platitudes. It demands an institutional reckoning. We must match policy with physiology. We must stop confusing inevitability with neglect. Until our institutions align with biology, and our policies reflect the reality of fatigue, we will keep losing lives, not just to sleep loss, but to a system that treats exhaustion as a footnote instead of a warning flare.

This book exists to challenge that inertia. To speak for those whose biology is breaking under the weight of silence, and to offer a path forward that doesn't rest just on the shoulders of the exhausted.

The Parking Lot Pause: 3 Steps Before You Drive

Why it matters:

Fatigue doesn't wait until the highway. Research shows the first signs of impairment can appear within **15 minutes** of leaving work. The Parking Lot Pause gives your biology a buffer before the drive home.

Step 1: Stop

Don't rush straight to the car.

Find a safe, quiet space (a recovery room if available, or stay parked).

Step 2: Reset (10–20 minutes)

Choose one:

Nap: A brief "parking lot nap" (10–20 minutes) can restore alertness.

Hydrate: Drink water to counter fatigue and dehydration.

Light control: Use sunglasses if driving home in daylight, or expose yourself to bright light if you need to stay awake.

Optional: Take safe, low-risk aids (e.g., glycine an hour before intended sleep at home).

Step 3: Go

Once you feel alert, start the drive.

If you're still drowsy, don't risk it. Use rideshare, carpool, or public transit if possible.

Key Principle:

Your shift isn't over until you arrive home safely. Treat the commute as part of the job. A 15-minute pause could be the most important thing you do all day.

Clock Notes

Microsleep: A brief, involuntary episode of sleep lasting only a few seconds. It often occurs without warning in severely sleep-deprived individuals, especially during monotonous tasks like driving home after a night shift.

Drowsy Driving: Operating a vehicle while cognitively impaired due to lack of sleep. For shift workers, this impairment can mirror or exceed the effects of alcohol, and often strikes within minutes of leaving the workplace parking lot.

Fatigue Impairment Curve: A pattern in which cognitive and motor function decline rapidly with sustained wakefulness. Studies show significant driving deterioration within 15 minutes post-shift, with near-crash events peaking after 45 minutes.

Systemic Outcome: A consequence not of individual error, but of larger institutional design. These crashes are not flukes—they are the predictable result of biology ignored by scheduling norms.

Circadian Collision: The mismatch between biological night and social demands (like a commute after a night shift). This collision amplifies risk, slows reaction time, and makes fatigue unavoidable, not optional.

The Biological Price Tag

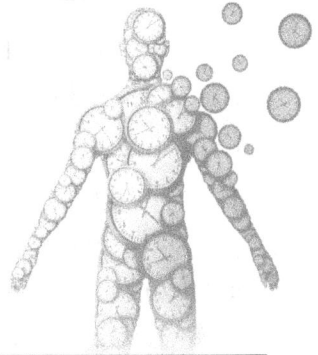

The world doesn't stop.

It runs on demand, fueled by a 24/7 economy built to deliver everything instantly. We've accepted this perpetual motion as normal, even inevitable. Technology sustains the illusion of convenience, of seamless continuity. *But at what cost?*

This chapter pulls back the curtain on that cost. It reveals the biological toll of a 24/7 society, and why your health is quietly traded every time the clock dictates.

Behind the grind of our 24/7 world is a hidden workforce, the human capital that keeps the machine running while the rest of the world sleeps. And that machine extracts something precious in return.

And the cost isn't financial. It's paid in biological currency: broken sleep, hormonal chaos, cognitive fatigue, and the slow erosion of systems never designed to run in darkness.

This isn't metaphor. It's measurable—in mitochondria, in blood pressure spikes, in metabolic collapse. It isn't just a toll. It's a transaction. One body at a time.

Night after night, while the rest of the world sleeps, millions of workers clock in. In the United States alone, 16% of all wage and salary workers operate outside the bounds of a typical 9-to-5 schedule.[5] They are the lifeblood of our society, staffing hospitals, stocking shelves, safeguarding communities, and running the infrastructure that never stops. But beneath the glow of fluorescent lights and the hum of late-night productivity lies a grim biological reality: for many, their work is a slow-motion assault on their health.

One of the most immediate consequences is a diagnosable condition known as shift work sleep disorder (SWSD). It's not just feeling tired. The official medical definition describes a debilitating pattern of excessive sleepiness and insomnia that lasts for at least a month, directly impairing a person's ability to function at work and in their personal life.[6] It is the clinical name for a body at war with its own internal clock, a clock that has been thrown into chaos by a work schedule.

This book is not a scientific treatise designed to dispute decades of research. It's a bridge. This is where your transformation begins: not by escaping shift work, but by understanding its invisible toll, and learning how to fight back from the inside out. It connects the established science of human health with the lived reality of those whose biology is under siege: the shift workers, the night laborers, the people holding society together while their own systems unravel.

We will lean into the science, not to overwhelm, but to empower. Because understanding *why* shift work breaks the body is the first, most critical step to reclaiming your health.

My purpose is twofold: First, to arm you with a clear understanding of the physiological toll this schedule imposes. Second, to show you exactly where your power lies: in the choices you make, the rhythms you protect, and the environment you shape.

You cannot change the system overnight. But you can change your strategy. And sometimes, that's the difference between erosion and resilience.

At the heart of this entire discussion is one core concept: circadian disruption.

In 2007, this concept was thrust into the global spotlight. The International Agency for Research on Cancer (IARC), a specialized branch of the World Health Organization (WHO), delivered a landmark classification. It declared that shift work involving circadian disruption is "probably carcinogenic to humans" (Group 2A).[7] This wasn't a guess; it was a conclusion based on sufficient evidence from animal studies and limited, but deeply concerning, data in humans.

Proving that shift work directly causes cancer is notoriously difficult.

The life of a shift worker is a perfect storm of overlapping risk. Poor diet, reduced physical activity, and higher rates of smoking or alcohol use are often part of the landscape. Add to that the chronic sleep deprivation and elevated stress that define this lifestyle, and you begin to see the web: a dense tangle of biological strain.

Then layer in the occupational hazards: exposure to radiation, industrial chemicals, diesel fumes, or night-after-night emotional trauma. Healthcare. Manufacturing. Transportation. These jobs don't just break the clock—they break the body.

And so the science struggles. Isolating circadian disruption as the singular cause is nearly impossible, because in a shift worker's world, nothing is isolated.

This is why the current body of human research, while showing a clear *association* between shift work and cancer, stops short of proving direct causation. But in controlled animal studies where those confounding factors are stripped away, the evidence is undeniable: disrupting the circadian rhythm has a clear carcinogenic effect.[8] This is what scientists call "biological plausibility." It's the smoking gun that gives the IARC's classification its weight and urgency. And it leads to a powerful conclusion: even if we can't prove causation in humans yet, any effort to reduce circadian disruption for shift workers is a rational, evidence-based strategy to lower their long-term health risks.

So, what does it mean to be a "probable carcinogen"? Where does shift work stand in the scientific landscape of risk? It resides in the same toxic neighborhood as some well-known threats. The Group 2A list includes industrial chemicals like acrylamide and lead compounds; emissions from high-temperature frying; the consumption of red meat; and drinking beverages hotter than 149°F (65°C). That list also includes chemotherapy drugs, specific viruses like HPV type 68, and even malaria.[7]

The fact that shift work sits alongside carcinogens isn't alarmist—it's clarity.

It's a signal to take circadian disruption seriously. The damage from a misaligned sleep-wake cycle may be less visible than a chemical exposure, but the biological consequences are just as real, and just as measurable.

This classification doesn't sensationalize the risk. It contextualizes it. And it gives us the rationale to treat disrupted sleep not as a lifestyle inconvenience, but as a legitimate occupational hazard.

Of all the threats shift workers face, one towers above the rest: the chronic lack of restorative sleep.[9] It is the most significant variable and often the most difficult to control. But before we can find solutions, we must first truly understand the problem. The science must be made accessible, so that those who are most affected can build a foundation of knowledge. Only then can we empower informed choices and implement the small, impactful changes that lead to better health.

For some, the culture of shift work is part of the appeal.

The night shift offers autonomy, fewer interruptions, and a rhythm that feels quieter, more focused. It suits the independent, the introverted, the adaptable. It can serve a lifestyle that demands flexibility—raising children, pursuing education, or simply avoiding the chaos of the day.

But this is the paradox's cruelest trick: personal preference does not override human physiology. You may love the night shift. You may thrive in its quiet. But your biology isn't participating in the choice.

Circadian disruption doesn't wait for symptoms. It unfolds in silence, beneath the surface, behind the scenes, regardless of how you *feel*. Knowledge isn't just power—it's protection. And in a world where the damage is invisible until it isn't, protection is everything.

Clock Notes

Circadian Disruption – The breakdown of the body's natural biological rhythm due to misaligned sleep-wake cycles; central to the health consequences of shift work.

Shift Work Sleep Disorder (SWSD) – A diagnosable condition characterized by chronic insomnia and excessive sleepiness directly linked to irregular shift schedules.

Biological Plausibility – The scientific rationale connecting circadian disruption with long-term disease risk, including cancer, even when causation is hard to prove in human studies.

Group 2A Carcinogen – The World Health Organization's classification of shift work involving circadian disruption as "probably carcinogenic to humans," alongside lead, acrylamide, and high-temp cooking emissions.

Restorative Sleep – Deep, undisturbed sleep that supports immune function, cellular repair, and metabolic health, often sacrificed in shift workers due to misaligned schedules.

Ancient Rhythms and Contemporary Challenges

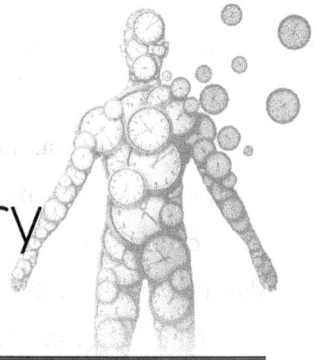

Shift work didn't begin with the modern world.

It is an ancient practice, born from something deeply primal: the need for protection. Long before factories and fluorescent lights, there were watchers in the dark—nomadic shepherds, tribal sentinels, fire-keepers—those who stayed awake while others slept, their torches pushing back against the night.

They weren't driven by productivity. They were driven by survival. But over time, survival gave way to production. And what began as protection turned into a cycle of exploitation, one that still runs under the surface of today's economy. Understanding where shift work began is essential to reclaiming your place within it. The first shift workers weren't managing output. They were guarding life.

In ancient Rome, that primal duty became a profession.

It was formalized in one of history's first organized shift-based workforces: the *Vigiles*, a hybrid of firefighters and law enforcers who patrolled the city through the night.[10] Their shifts followed the arc of the sun and the pulse of the city.

They were Rome's guardians, awake while others slept, tasked with holding back the chaos of darkness.

For millennia, night work was a necessity, but a limited one.

It served survival, not scale. That changed with the Industrial Revolution. It was here that our appetite for around-the-clock production was born—and with it, a new kind of exhaustion.

Long before Thomas Edison's incandescent bulb flooded the darkness in 1879, the gears of industry were already turning through the night. Textile mills churned. Coal mines groaned. Workers labored in 24-hour shifts beneath the dim glow of candles and oil lamps, their bodies pushed beyond the rhythms they were built to follow. [11]

It was no longer about protection. It was about profit.

The blueprint for modern exploitation was drafted in the 1820s in Lowell, Massachusetts. There, a planned textile manufacturing town rose from the ground, built on a system of integrated production that would be replicated across New England. The engine of this system was a workforce of an estimated 8,000 'mill girls': young, marginalized women and children recruited from rural farming backgrounds to operate the deafening looms and machinery.[12] They were chosen for a simple, brutal reason: they would accept lower wages and offer less resistance.

This is the legacy of shift work: resistance—and exploitation.

The faces have changed. The industries have evolved. But the pattern remains. What once lived in the contracts of mill girls now lives in the algorithms of modern scheduling software.

Dangerously long hours. Hazardous conditions. Economic vulnerability.

The same critiques that haunted 19th-century factories still echo across hospitals, warehouses, and overnight routes today.

The machines may be faster and the lights brighter, but the biology, and the burden, remain the same.

The industries have evolved, but the biology hasn't. The forces that once shaped life in coal mines and textile mills still echo in hospital wards and delivery routes. This isn't just history, it's a blueprint for understanding why the system still demands more than the body can give. Modern shift workers are still concentrated in sectors with precarious protections: healthcare, manufacturing, hospitality, and transportation.[13]

Demographics tell the story starkly. Today, women still fill a disproportionate number of night shift roles. Education is a powerful determinant, with nearly 20% of individuals lacking a high school diploma working non-day shifts, a far higher rate than their more educated peers.[14] Income inequality is just as glaring: over 21% of workers in the lowest income bracket work nights, compared to just 8.3% in the highest bracket.[14]

This burden extends far beyond the workplace.

It seeps into relationships, routines, and the quiet architecture of daily life. It breeds a particular kind of isolation—not just physical, but temporal. A life lived out of sync.

While the world sleeps, they work.

While families gather, they recover.

Birthdays are missed. Weekends vanish. Morning becomes night. Holidays arrive like static through a broken signal.

This isn't just social inconvenience—it's social disconnection.

A slow, quiet erosion of belonging.

But the most devastating cost is physiological. More than half of all work shifts actively disrupt our circadian rhythms, whether through night schedules, quick returns between shifts, or extended hours. And while we tend to focus on the night shift, even early morning and evening schedules misalign the body's clock, chipping away at worker well-being.[15]

The scientific literature is unequivocal, linking these non-standard schedules to a cascade of chronic diseases: cardiovascular disease, workplace injury, hypertension, breast cancer, metabolic disorders, and diabetes.[16,17]

Within the complex interplay of nutrition, movement, and medicine, one truth rises above the rest. Sleep is the body's most essential, non-negotiable biological process.[18]

And for shift workers, it's the one we willingly sacrifice.

By defying the body's most ancient and essential rhythm, modern shift work has become one of the most unrelenting, and most overlooked, forces eroding our collective health. Not because sleep doesn't matter, but because the system demands we act like it doesn't.

Clock Notes

Social Desynchronization – Shift work creates not just sleep disruption, but time disruption. It erodes belonging by isolating workers from social rituals, family rhythms, and shared time zones.

Circadian Misalignment – Over half of all shift schedules today, including early morning and evening shifts, disrupt the body's internal clock, not just overnights.

Structural Inequality – Women, low-income earners, and individuals with limited education remain disproportionately represented in shift roles, bearing the biological and social brunt of around-the-clock labor.

Our Biochemical Pacemaker

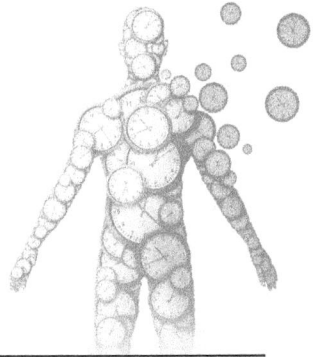

Beneath the glow of modern life, a deeper rhythm pulses—ancient, unyielding, and often ignored. This chapter brings that rhythm into focus. Not as metaphor but as literal machinery, coded deep in our biology.

Because if shift work breaks the body by disrupting time, then timing itself becomes your first and most powerful tool for repair.

It is ancient. Immutable.

Not shaped by technology or social expectation, but by the Earth's rotation on its axis, a legacy of evolution etched into the DNA of nearly every living thing.

From the fruit fly to the blue whale, from single-celled organisms to the most complex mammals, this internal 24-hour cycle is not optional.[19]

It is a biological constant. A law of life.

Though we haven't explored it fully, the consequences of disrupting this rhythm are far from trivial. Decades of research have drawn undeniable links between circadian misalignment and a host of modern diseases, including cardiovascular disease, obesity, diabetes, and depression.[20] While shift workers face the most extreme and chronic form of this disruption, the reality is that our 24/7 culture has pushed most of us into some level of circadian dysfunction. To fight back, we must first understand the machinery.

At the center of our internal universe is a tiny, powerful cluster of nerve cells located in the hypothalamus of the brain: the suprachiasmatic nucleus, or SCN. [21] Think of it as our biochemical pacemaker or master clock. This is the central command that dictates the timing of our entire physiology.[21] This internal command center sets the circadian timing system. But how does it know what time it is in the world outside?

The answer is light. Light is the most critical timing cue—or zeitgeber, German for "time giver"—for the human body. When light enters our eyes, specialized light-sensitive cells in the retina containing melanopsin send a direct signal to the SCN, a pathway known as the retinohypothalamic tract.[22,23] This daily signal of dawn and dusk is what allows our master clock to synchronize itself with the local environment, anchoring our internal biology to the 24-hour day.

But the SCN is not the only clock in the body. It is the conductor of a vast orchestra of peripheral clocks, located in our liver, gut, muscles, and nearly every other organ system.[24] The SCN sends out signals to keep this orchestra in sync, ensuring all our bodily functions are playing from the same sheet of music.

This is where a second, powerful zeitgeber enters the scene: food.

While light sets the master clock in the brain, the timing of our meals speaks directly to the peripheral clocks, especially in the liver, pancreas, and gut. [25] These metabolic clocks are exquisitely sensitive to when we eat, not just what we eat.

Rhythmic feeding, eating during our biological daytime, amplifies the signal from the SCN, keeping the entire circadian system in harmony. When light and food are aligned, the body hums in coherence. When they're out of sync, even the best diet can become a source of internal confusion.

Here, we arrive at the heart of the problem for the shift worker.

Working through the night means eating during the body's designated rest phase. And that single act, eating at biological midnight, sends a powerful, contradictory signal to your internal clocks.

The peripheral clocks in your liver and gut are hearing one message: *It's daytime—digest, metabolize, store energy.*

But your master clock, still loosely tethered to the light-dark cycle, is whispering the opposite: *It's night—rest, repair, shut down.*

The result is desynchronization.

The orchestra falls out of tune. The liver clock drifts away from the brain's conductor.

And in that internal discord, systems falter.

Hormones misfire. Metabolism stumbles.

This is not just theory—it's the biological chaos that fuels the chronic disease patterns we see in shift workers every day. [26]

Understanding this mechanism is crucial.

It reveals that the harm of shift work isn't just about lost sleep—it's about systemic misalignment. A full-body desynchronization that affects not just rest, but metabolism, mood, immunity, and long-term health.

But within that disruption lies a clue.

If the body runs on time, then timing itself becomes a tool.

By understanding how our clocks keep rhythm, we can begin to realign—not perfectly, but meaningfully—toward a life that runs with biology, not against it.

Clock Notes

Suprachiasmatic Nucleus (SCN) – The brain's master clock, located in the hypothalamus, that regulates nearly every biological rhythm in the body using light as its primary timing cue.

Zeitgeber – A German term meaning "time giver," referring to environmental signals, like light and food, that synchronize our internal clocks with the external world.

Peripheral Clocks – Independent biological clocks found in organs like the liver, gut, and muscles, which rely on cues such as food timing to stay aligned with the SCN.

Desynchronization – A breakdown in internal harmony when the body's master and peripheral clocks receive conflicting cues, such as eating at night, leading to metabolic and hormonal dysfunction.

Rhythmic Feeding – Aligning meal timing with the body's natural daytime phase to support circadian coherence and prevent the internal chaos triggered by night-eating.: Lessons from Ancient Algae.

The Oldest Clock
on Earth

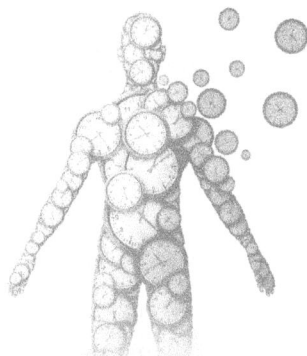

To understand the modern crisis of shift work, we have to go back billions of years to one of Earth's simplest organisms: blue-green algae.

In the study of a microscopic cyanobacterium called *Synechococcus elongatus*, scientists discovered something profound: even this ancient, single-celled organism runs on a clock.[27]

And when that clock is aligned with its environment, it thrives. When it's misaligned, it falters.

This isn't just microbial trivia. It's a foundational principle that echoes across all life, including us.

Life functions best when it is in rhythm with its surroundings. This chapter takes us back to the source, to the first organisms that evolved in sync with the sun, and forward to the strategies you can use to re-align your own system. Because if algae can evolve to survive by mastering light, so can you. And when that rhythm breaks, so does everything else.

This humble, photosynthetic bacterium, found in oceans and lakes across the globe, possesses a fully functional circadian clock.[28] In the 1990s, this discovery was revolutionary. Scientists proved that this intricate timekeeping ability, once thought to be exclusive to complex organisms (eukaryotes), was present in some of the planet's earliest and simplest life forms (prokaryotes). *S. elongatus* doesn't just have a clock—it depends on it for survival. It anticipates the rising and setting of the sun, optimizing essential functions like photosynthesis and nitrogen fixation to gain a decisive advantage. This is not just a quaint biological feature; it is an evolutionary mandate, the very foundation of circadian biology.

But this understanding didn't begin with cyanobacteria. The earliest recorded observation of daily rhythmic behavior comes from Androsthenes of Thasos in the fourth century BCE, who described the diurnal leaf movements of the tamarind tree.[29] Nearly two millennia later, in 1729, French physicist Jean-Jacques d'Ortus de Mairan observed the same rhythmic leaf movements in *Mimosa pudica*, even when the plant was kept in total darkness, proving the existence of an internal clock.[30] Since then, circadian rhythms have been found in nearly every kingdom of life: in the pupal eclosion of *Drosophila*, the wheel-running behavior of mice, and the sleep-wake cycles of humans.[28]

Recent advances in circadian cell biology have further confirmed that these rhythms are not abstract patterns—they are encoded at the molecular level, governed by feedback loops involving core clock genes like PER, CRY, and CLOCK.[31] These molecular rhythms operate autonomously in nearly every cell, forming the invisible scaffolding that organizes life across all species.

The same principles that govern this ancient algae also govern us.

The word *circadian* comes from the Latin *circa* ("around") and *dies* ("day"), a rhythm that repeats roughly every 24 hours.[32] And this rhythm isn't random. It's defined by three key properties that appear across almost all forms of life.

First, the rhythm persists even without external cues. It keeps oscillating on its own, even in total darkness.

Second, it's temperature-compensated, holding steady even when the environment heats up or cools down. And third, and most importantly, it can be entrained.

It can be synchronized by signals from the outside world. Chief among them: light and dark.[33] This ability to sync with the environment is not just biological convenience—it's biological necessity. It's what keeps our bodies in step with the world we live in.

This is where the lesson from ancient algae becomes a practical strategy for the modern shift worker. The same environmental cues that guide *S. elongatus* can be leveraged to protect human biology from the consequences of a misaligned schedule.

For night shift workers, this means learning how to use light as a tool, not just passively, but strategically.

Bright, controlled light exposure before and during the shift can enhance alertness, performance, and circadian adaptation.[34]

Just as critically, exposure to natural morning light, especially during the commute home, must be minimized. Wear sunglasses. Use blackout curtains. Create a cave-like sleep environment.

Because even a few minutes of bright light at the wrong time can reset the master clock, robbing you of the deep, restorative sleep your biology is already fighting to preserve.[35]

Beyond these immediate strategies lies something deeper: the power of understanding the science itself.

A list of tips can solve a problem for a day. But understanding the *why* builds a skill for a lifetime.

When you realize that your body is governed by the same ancient, light-sensitive biology as blue-green algae, you gain more than knowledge—you gain leverage.

You gain the ability to adapt, troubleshoot, and refine your approach no matter how your schedule shifts, or how many times your life is turned upside down.

When you understand how your biology works, you stop guessing. You start choosing with intention, and that changes everything.

Clock Notes

Synechococcus elongatus – A single-celled cyanobacterium that possesses a circadian clock, demonstrating that even Earth's earliest life forms evolved with biological timing systems.

Circadian Rhythm – A ~24-hour internal cycle found across nearly all life forms, governing essential processes like sleep, metabolism, and cellular repair.

Entrainment – The ability of biological clocks to synchronize with environmental cues, primarily light and darkness, ensuring alignment with the external world.

The Shift Worker's Creed

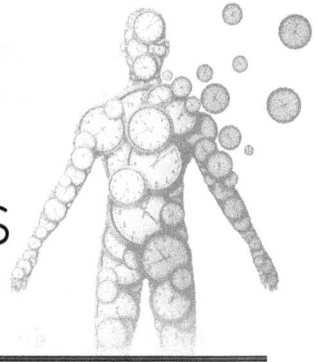

Let's pause for a moment.

The first chapters of this book were built around systems—metabolic clocks, historical injustice, biological pathways, circadian breakdown. And for good reason: you can't navigate a problem until you understand the terrain. But sometimes, after mapping out the physiology, you have to stop and ask: *What does it feel like to live here?*

That's what this chapter is.

I wanted to address psychological well-being because it holds enormous value—and because too many shift workers are medicated, depressed, or silently suffering. Not just struggling, but *unseen* in that struggle. Performing under pressure while slowly unraveling behind the scenes.

We don't talk about it enough. And when we do, it's often flattened into self-care slogans or wellness checklists. That's not what this chapter is.

This is about what it really takes to protect yourself while working a schedule that was never designed for human biology. It's about what I've seen, what I've lived, and what I believe can help you survive it too.

Let me be clear: I'm not a mental health professional. I'm not a psychiatrist, psychologist, or therapist. I'm a nurse who has spent over

30 years in the field, many of those on the night shift. I've seen what humans can do to each other, and to themselves. I've done things to myself, and to others, that I'm not proud of.

You don't survive decades in this profession without carrying what it leaves behind.

And I understand how bad it can get. I'm not writing this from some polished version of myself. I believe I suffer from a degree of high-functioning depression—just well enough to keep showing up, but not well enough to feel truly restored. And I know I'm not alone.

When you are a shift worker, the damage runs deep, and you won't recover with one or two basic tweaks. You will have to work hard to protect yourself.

It's going to require significant changes, not because you're flawed, but because you're up against something big. And we don't defeat big challenges with small adjustments.

As a veteran of shift work, I know exactly what produces poor outcomes because I've lived them. I've also learned what makes me feel a little less miserable. What eases the mental crash.

This chapter is a reflection on a decade spent in the trenches, on what keeps the wheels turning when everything else is falling apart. I don't think I'm unique. I believe these processes will work for you too.

Shift workers are different.

And yet, the world still expects us to perform. To keep families intact, show up for overtime shifts, drive home without crashing, and somehow maintain a stable identity through it all.

We live with constant physiological, psychological, and social obstacles that can't be managed like a side hustle. It's not something we can address "when we have time." That time rarely comes.

Instead, we need a framework, a set of behaviors and boundaries that are non-negotiable, even on the hardest days.

One of the core tenets of this book is that your overall health depends on understanding the underlying rhythms of your biology. That includes your mind. Psychological well-being isn't just about mindset; it's shaped by biology. Mood, motivation, focus—they rise and fall with your rhythms. You can't separate mental health from the body that sustains it.

As we've already established, your biology runs on rhythm. Every major system in your body—your heart, your gut, your liver, your immune system—follows a timing pattern. These aren't random processes. They're synchronized cycles, calibrated to light, food, and sleep.

Disrupt the rhythm, and you disrupt the system.

Your brain is no different.

It doesn't float above the body—it depends on it.

It needs sleep, blood flow, oxygen, and energy. Without those inputs, it doesn't prioritize joy or calm. It prioritizes survival.

When that rhythm breaks, everything else begins to fall apart.

You can't outthink a sleep-deprived brain.

If you don't check the basic boxes—biological, psychological, and social, in that order—shift work will break you down. Slowly. Quietly. Eventually.

You are the architect, and the advocate, for your own recovery.

At some point, you have to name the challenge.

Say it out loud: "I am a shift worker."

Not as an excuse. Not as a badge of martyrdom. As a strategy.

"I am a shift worker, and these are the behaviors I need to manage my life as a shift worker."

That's where your agency lives. In accepting the challenge, and doing the work.

That means saying: *This is who I am. This is the life I live. These are the behaviors I need to survive it.*

You can't wait until you feel like it. That day won't come.

This book will return again and again to one idea: A small range of well-researched, repeatable behaviors will get you through.

Frame it this way.

If you wanted to destroy your health, what would you do?

You'd stay up all night. Eat at inconsistent times. Skip exercise. Avoid people. Rely on caffeine. Sleep when you crash. Let your emotions run unchecked. Neglect your social environment.

That's what many shift workers do, because the job demands it.

Now do the opposite.

You don't have to get everything right. You don't even have to start big.

But you do have to start on purpose.

Psychological wellness isn't just for crises. It's for Tuesday at 4 p.m. It's for the normal, average days, because that's what most of life is. Your well-being lives in the tiny, repetitive acts: walking instead of scrolling, prepping one meal, skipping the extra caffeine, sending a text instead of ghosting a friend.

The relationship you have with yourself is the most important one you'll ever maintain. Your voice, the one inside your head, is the one you hear the most.

Make it honest.

Make it strong.

Make it yours.

The Shift Worker's Creed

I will stop borrowing from the 9-to-5 world and expecting it to fit my reality.

I will own the fact that I am a shift worker, and build my life around it, not against it.

I will be the architect of my health, not its hostage.

I will build habits that hold on ordinary days, not just ideal ones. I will move, eat, sleep, and recover in rhythm with my biology, because lasting health begins with alignment.

I will accept that without a process, there are consequences—and I choose to lead, not react.

Let's get to work.

The Hidden Metabolic Gatekeepers

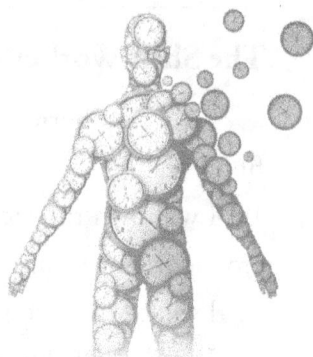

Misalignment isn't a metaphor—it's a mechanism. Studies in both humans and animals have shown that when circadian rhythms are disrupted, insulin resistance rises.[36] Blood pressure creeps up. Inflammatory markers spike.[37] Over time, this cascade of dysregulation leads to the hallmarks of metabolic syndrome: elevated fasting glucose, increased waist circumference, high triglycerides, and low HDL cholesterol.[36]

When the clocks drift apart, the rhythms unravel. It's like trying to play jazz with a broken metronome. They tell your gut when to absorb nutrients, your pancreas when to release insulin, your liver when to store or mobilize energy.

While the brain's master clock sets the rhythm for our daily lives, the real metabolic work happens locally, deep within the tissues of the body. Here, a vast network of peripheral clocks operates silently, behind the scenes.

They are the hidden timekeepers of the gut, liver, pancreas, muscle, and fat—gatekeepers of energy, guardians of balance. This chapter pulls back the curtain on the body's internal command structure, where local clocks oversee high-stakes operations in digestion, insulin control, and cellular metabolism. Their breakdown isn't just biology—it's your blueprint for reclaiming order.

And when they fall out of sync with the master clock, or with each other, the consequences ripple outward: confusion, inefficiency, and eventually, disease.

So where does this breakdown begin? With the clocks themselves. Let's take a closer look at the roles of these metabolic gatekeepers.

The peripheral clocks in the liver, pancreas, and adipose (fat) tissue operate in a semi-autonomous way—responding to local cues like nutrient intake, insulin, and energy demand—while still taking orders from the brain's master clock.[38]

It's a dual command structure: central coordination, local execution. And when those signals conflict, the result is confusion—metabolic chaos at the cellular level. In adipose tissue, these clocks regulate fat storage and release. When misaligned, they can promote fat accumulation, increasing the risk of obesity.[39] Fat cells, long thought of as mere storage, are endocrine players that communicate via hormones like leptin.[40]

The liver's internal clock governs gluconeogenesis and lipid metabolism; when disrupted, glucose homeostasis collapses, contributing to insulin resistance and fatty liver disease.[39]

Skeletal muscle, a major site for glucose uptake, becomes less responsive to insulin when its clock is out of sync, worsening glucose intolerance and fatigue. Even the gut microbiome, once thought of as a passive resident, adheres to circadian rhythms. Disrupted sleep and meal timing shift microbial composition—promoting inflammation, impairing digestion, and disturbing energy regulation.[41]

Even in tightly controlled lab studies, simulating shift work without any added stressors, researchers have observed measurable harm—glucose intolerance and reduced insulin sensitivity, sometimes within days.[42]

Misalignment between the central and peripheral clocks doesn't just create inefficiency; it creates vulnerability. Metabolic, cognitive, immunologic.

It breeds pathology.

Even minor misalignments, like those caused by daylight saving time, can nudge this system off course. Living on the western edge of a time zone, for example, may increase your risk of diabetes and cardiovascular disease simply because the behavioral cues (like work start times) are misaligned with solar time.[43]

For the shift worker, this is where the biological conflict becomes intensely personal. The constant state of circadian misalignment—working when the body expects rest, eating when it expects to fast—unleashes chaos on these peripheral clocks. The rhythmic fluctuation of metabolites in our blood and tissues, a process honed by evolution to optimize energy use, is thrown into disarray.[44] The body's finely tuned sensitivity to insulin and its ability to manage blood sugar, which naturally shift throughout a 24-hour cycle, become dangerously unstable.[45]

This creates a devastating biological feedback loop. We now understand that the relationship between clock dysfunction and metabolic stress is bidirectional. A disrupted schedule impairs metabolic regulation, and in turn, the resulting metabolic imbalance further destabilizes the clocks. It is a vicious cycle that accelerates the path toward chronic disease.

When these local managers receive conflicting signals—light from the eyes says it's night, but food in the stomach says it's daytime—the system begins to falter.

Confusion at the cellular level leads to dysfunction at the whole-body level.

Understanding this internal conflict is the key.

It moves us beyond the vague idea that shift work is "unhealthy" and into a precise understanding of the biological battle being waged beneath the surface.

And it's from that foundation that real strategy emerges: targeted, evidence-based approaches designed to protect these vital metabolic gatekeepers, restore internal order, and break the cycle of misalignment and disease.

Because once you understand the conflict, you're no longer a passive participant in the damage. You're part of the repair

Clock Notes

Bidirectional Feedback Loop - The mutual reinforcement between circadian disruption and metabolic dysfunction—each worsening the other.

Dual Command Structure - The coordination system between the central clock (in the brain) and peripheral clocks (in tissues), requiring synchronized inputs to maintain balance.

Metabolic Chaos - The downstream effect of desynchronized clocks: impaired insulin signaling, glucose intolerance, fat accumulation, and chronic disease risk.

Peripheral Clocks – Tissue-specific timekeepers in the liver, pancreas, muscle, fat, and gut that regulate critical functions like insulin release, digestion, and nutrient metabolism.

β-Cell Failure and the Rise of Diabetes

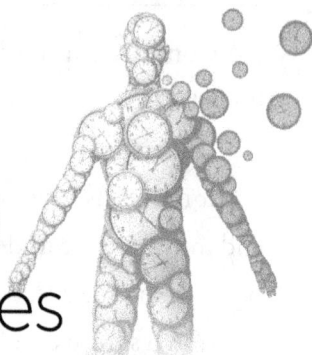

Imagine the β-cells deep inside your pancreas as an elite, microscopic emergency response team. Their sole mission? To manage your blood sugar, rushing to the scene after every meal to deploy insulin with precision and speed.

This chapter brings you inside the metabolic command center, where every mistimed bite, every sleepless night, becomes a signal. This isn't just blood sugar—it's cellular survival. And understanding this frontline gives you the power to defend it.

This team isn't just highly skilled. It's highly disciplined, operating on a tight 24-hour schedule set by your circadian rhythm.

But what happens when the emergency calls never stop? What happens when the timing is unpredictable, the shifts never end, and the schedule descends into chaos?

Eventually, even the best team breaks down. They lose their timing. They lose their accuracy. And what they fail to catch—glucose—builds up in the bloodstream, setting the stage for metabolic disease.

For the shift worker, this is not a theoretical exercise. This is the daily reality for their pancreatic β-cells. The constant state of circadian misalignment—the erratic eating, the disrupted sleep, the chronic inflammation—acts as a relentless barrage of stress signals. Over time, this assault leads to β-cell dysfunction, a silent and dangerous tipping point where the body's ability to manage glucose begins to break down.[46] This is the physiological point of no return, where insulin resistance cascades into full-blown type 2 diabetes.

The evidence linking shift work to this tipping point is now overwhelming. Numerous human studies have established a powerful association between prolonged shift work and an increased risk of developing type 2 diabetes.[47] Controlled clinical trials have demonstrated that even acute, short-term circadian misalignment, the kind experienced over just a few night shifts, is enough to dysregulate glucose homeostasis and impair the function of β-cells.[48]

The mechanism of this damage is rooted in the cell's own internal clock. β-cells possess an intrinsic circadian rhythm that governs their function, a rhythm that is meant to be synchronized with the master clock in the brain.[49] When circadian disruption occurs, this elegant system is compromised. The cells are flooded with oxidative stress, a surge of damaging molecules called reactive oxygen species—ROS—the cellular equivalent of biochemical shrapnel.[50] This relentless oxidative damage impairs the β-cells' ability to secrete insulin, eventually leading to their failure.[46]

And here lies the paradox—and the opportunity. You may not be able to change your work hours. But you *can* influence how your body's frontline responders, your β-cells, handle the pressure. Through the science of chrononutrition, strategic fasting, and targeted antioxidant support, we now have a toolkit to protect β-cell health in even the most chaotic schedules.

By avoiding high-glycemic meals during your circadian low, and anchoring your eating window to your true biological daytime, you can reduce the metabolic strain placed on your pancreas, right when it matters most.[51] Because preserving the health and precision of your β-cells is not just important—it's critical. It's the last barrier between adaptation and disease.

The key to defusing the metabolic time bomb of shift work isn't perfection.

It's timing. And it starts with one informed choice at a time. You can't clock out of your job. But your β-cells never get that choice. Time your choices—so theirs don't time out.

Clock Notes

β-Cell Dysfunction – The breakdown of pancreatic β-cells responsible for insulin secretion, often triggered by chronic circadian misalignment, oxidative stress, and metabolic strain.

Reactive Oxygen Species (ROS) – Chemically reactive molecules that accumulate during cellular stress; excessive ROS damages β-cells and disrupts insulin signaling.

Glucose Homeostasis – The body's ability to maintain stable blood glucose levels, a function heavily regulated by β-cells activity and vulnerable to shift-related disruptions.

Chrononutrition – A strategy that aligns meal timing with circadian rhythms to optimize metabolic function and reduce stress on insulin-secreting β-cells.

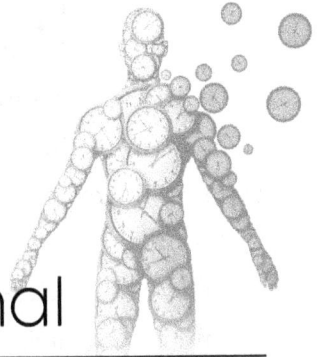

The Silenced Signal

The human body was never meant to digest darkness.

Our metabolism follows a rhythm, a daily cycle of fueling and fasting, hardwired by millions of years of evolution and governed by the rising and setting of the sun.

At the center of this ancient circuitry is a quiet but constant conversation, a metabolic dialogue between your fat cells and your brain. This chapter exposes what happens when that conversation breaks down. Not from weakness, but from misalignment. Because if your body can no longer hear its own signals, hunger becomes a whisper—and disease becomes the echo. And the moderator of that conversation is one of the body's most powerful hormones: leptin.

Leptin is the body's primary satiety signal; its job is to tell the brain, "We're full. You can stop eating now."

Like every other critical function, leptin secretion follows a strict circadian rhythm. [52] Its levels naturally rise in the evening and peak overnight, suppressing hunger and conserving energy while we sleep.[52] But for the shift worker, this elegant system is thrown into chaos. When night becomes day and meals arrive at biologically inappropriate times, the body's internal timekeeping goes haywire.[53]

The result is a dangerous feedback loop. Disrupted sleep-wake cycles flatten the natural peaks and valleys of leptin, dulling the body's ability to recognize when it's full.[54] This isn't about willpower. It's a failure of internal signaling, where clock genes like CLOCK and C/EBPα fall out of sync and the message gets scrambled.[55,56]

This chronic circadian disruption eventually leads to a perilous condition known as leptin resistance.[57] The body, in a desperate attempt to be heard, may even produce more leptin, but the brain's appetite-control centers in the hypothalamus no longer respond to the signal.[58] It's like shouting into a dead phone line. The body is sending the "I'm full" message, but the brain simply can't hear it.

This hormonal deafness has predictable and devastating consequences, promoting the overeating and late-night snacking that are so common among long-term shift workers.[59]

That creeping sense that you're no longer in control of your appetite isn't a failure of willpower—it's a failure of communication.

A breakdown in one of your body's most essential signaling systems: the link between your fat cells and your brain.

And it's not your fault. It's physiology. It's what happens when circadian rhythms fracture and hormones fall out of sync.

But understanding this breakdown is the first step toward repair.

It's how you begin to restore the connection, and reclaim control over your metabolic health. But to understand how far this system can fall, and what's left to salvage, we need to go deeper. There was a moment in science when leptin looked like the answer.

The miracle molecule.

The key to hunger, weight, metabolism—all of it.

Leptin isn't obscure. It's not niche. It's made by your own fat cells, released into your bloodstream like a chemical dispatch to the brain.

Because when the body stops listening to itself, hunger is no longer just a feeling. It's a symptom of metabolic confusion.

Its message?

We're full. We have enough. Turn down the appetite. Burn a little more.

It was meant to be self-regulating, an internal thermostat for energy. The more fat you had, the louder the leptin signal. In theory, this should've closed the loop: high fat → high leptin → less hunger → lower fat.

In theory.

But in practice, something broke.

The people with the *most* leptin—those living with obesity, type 2 diabetes, or fatty liver disease—weren't responding.[60] Their bodies were flooded with the signal. But their brains were deaf to it.

This is leptin resistance. And it changed everything.

The same hormone that should have quieted appetite and fueled energy expenditure was now whispering into static.

The speaker was on. The message was clear. The system just wasn't listening.

To understand what leptin *can* do, you have to see both versions of its story.

In rare cases—genetic mutations, extreme calorie deficits, or conditions like generalized and partial lipodystrophy—leptin levels drop dangerously low.[61] And when they do, the consequences are vast.

But here's the good news: replacement works. Administering leptin in these situations doesn't just help—it transforms.

- It shrinks fat mass.

- It boosts insulin sensitivity and lowers triglycerides.

- It repairs hormone systems, especially reproductive function.

- It supports immunity and strengthens bone.

This is leptin as a biological lifeline.

Now flip the script.

In most people struggling with metabolic disease, leptin is abundant, but the body is numb to it. More hormone won't help. It's like flooding a broken engine with gas.

The leptin is there. But the receptors aren't responding.

The signal is lost in the noise.

That's where we are now—standing at the edge of a system that made perfect biological sense... until modern life distorted the volume.

And for shift workers, that distortion is magnified.

Sleep disruption, circadian misalignment, inflammation, and erratic eating patterns all compound leptin resistance, making it harder to regulate hunger, satiety, and fat metabolism.[52]

Leptin hasn't failed. The environment has changed faster than evolution can adapt.

Scientists are now exploring ways to resensitize the brain to leptin, to break through the static. Animal studies are promising. Human trials are underway. But there's no silver bullet yet.

What remains is a profound biological insight: It's not just about how much leptin you have—it's about whether your body still knows how to listen.

And maybe that's the deeper lesson of shift work itself.

The rhythms, the signals, the conversations between systems, none of it disappears overnight.

But it does get quieter.

And when we stop listening to our own biology, disease isn't just possible.

It's inevitable.

Protect the signal. In a world built on noise, clarity is your greatest act of self-preservation.

Clock Notes

Leptin – A hormone secreted by fat cells that signals satiety to the brain. Its rhythmic release is disrupted by shift work, impairing the brain's ability to regulate appetite.

Leptin Resistance – A condition in which the brain becomes unresponsive to leptin's "I'm full" signal, leading to increased hunger and overeating despite elevated leptin levels.

Circadian Regulation of Appetite – The natural timing system that governs hunger and satiety, typically suppressing appetite overnight and reactivating it during the biological day.

CLOCK Protein – A core circadian gene involved in regulating metabolic and hormonal rhythms; disruption of CLOCK function contributes to miscommunication between fat cells and the brain.

Hypothalamic Signaling – The brain's central hub for interpreting hormonal cues related to hunger and fullness; impaired signaling in this region underlies appetite dysregulation in shift workers.

Microbial Rhythms and the Metabolic Toll

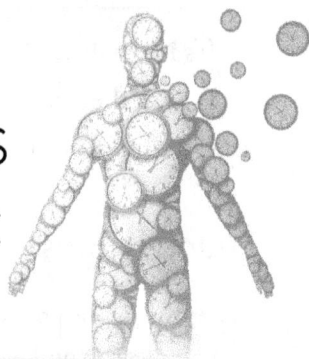

One of shift work's most invisible casualties hides in your gut, an ecosystem disrupted long before symptoms ever surface. And when its rhythms fracture, your metabolism pays the price.

Beneath the surface of every shift worker's routine—beneath the long hours, the skipped meals, the fractured sleep—there's a hidden ecosystem recording every disruption.

It doesn't sleep. It doesn't forget. And it never stops responding.

This is the gut microbiome: trillions of microbes living in your digestive tract, small but powerful regulators of your health.

Once dismissed as passive passengers, these microscopic organisms are now understood to be powerful regulators of metabolism, immunity, mood, even circadian rhythm itself.[62]

And when shift work scrambles your schedule, the microbiome feels it first.

We now know it acts as a critical inner sentinel, a second clock that synchronizes with the body's master circadian rhythm to regulate digestion, metabolism, and immunity.[63]

For a healthy individual, this internal ecosystem works in harmony with the body. But for the shift worker, it is thrown into a state of chronic disarray known as gut dysbiosis. The microbial allies that once supported health become saboteurs, altering hormone release, promoting inflammation, and sabotaging metabolic regulation.[64]

Like the human body itself, the gut microbiota operates on a strict 24-hour cycle.[62] The composition and activity of these intestinal bacteria fluctuate predictably throughout the day, driven by our feeding and fasting schedules. These microbial rhythms are essential for regulating our metabolism and energy balance. When a misaligned work schedule disrupts them, the consequences are severe, contributing directly to metabolic diseases like obesity, insulin resistance, and type 2 diabetes.[65]

Experimental studies show exactly how the damage unfolds. When the body's internal clock is disrupted, whether through genetic manipulation of core clock genes like BMAL1 or through simulated jet lag, the results are striking.[66]

Feeding patterns become erratic. The gut microbiome destabilizes.

And the downstream effects are immediate: impaired glucose tolerance, disrupted fat metabolism, and a measurable surge in inflammatory markers.[62]

In other words, the moment the clock breaks, the body begins to misfire, one system at a time. In short, a misaligned master clock creates a misaligned gut, which in turn poisons our metabolic health.[67]

This creates a perfect storm when combined with the hormonal shifts of sleep deprivation.

For the exhausted shift worker, levels of ghrelin, the "hunger hormone," tend to rise during the biological night, while leptin, the satiety hormone, declines.[68] This drives a powerful, hormonally charged urge to overeat precisely when the body is least prepared to handle the calories. At the same time, elevated levels of the stress hormone cortisol further impair insulin signaling and fuel systemic inflammation.[69]

This internal chaos is reflected in the very composition of the gut. Studies show that sleep restriction alters the gut microbiome in a specific way, increasing the ratio of Firmicutes to Bacteroidetes, a microbial signature strongly associated with obesity.[70] This distinct pattern has been observed in numerous shift-working populations, from healthcare providers to industrial laborers, linking their demanding schedules directly to a gut environment that promotes chronic disease.[71]

The gut microbiome is not a passive bystander—it's an active participant in the physiological fallout of shift work. When rhythms break, it responds. When patterns change, it changes with them.

But within that disruption lies opportunity. Because the gut is also remarkably responsive. It adapts quickly. It listens to timing, to diet, to environment.

And that means it can be retrained.

Early evidence strongly supports the use of targeted strategies like probiotic supplementation, precision nutritional timing, and rigorous sleep hygiene to fight dysbiosis, restore microbial rhythms, and build metabolic resilience.[72]

Clock Notes

Gut Microbiome – The vast community of microorganisms in the digestive tract that plays a central role in regulating metabolism, immune function, and circadian alignment.

Gut Dysbiosis – A microbial imbalance or maladaptation in the gut, often triggered by shift work, irregular eating, and disrupted sleep, leading to inflammation and metabolic dysfunction.

Microbial Rhythms – The circadian-like fluctuations in microbial composition and activity that regulate digestion, energy balance, and immune response; easily disrupted by misaligned schedules.

Firmicutes-to-Bacteroidetes Ratio – A commonly used biomarker of gut health; an increased ratio has been linked to obesity and is often elevated in shift workers experiencing circadian misalignment.

Ghrelin and Leptin Imbalance – Hormonal shifts during sleep loss and night work that increase hunger (via ghrelin) and suppress satiety (via leptin), compounding the effects of microbial disruption.

Interlude: What Aristotle Knew That Shift Workers Forget

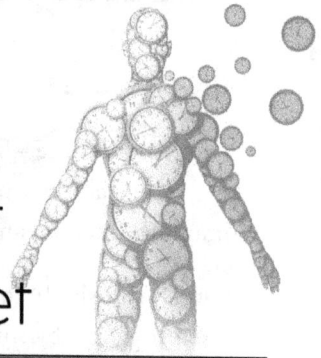

The hardest part of change isn't knowledge. It's action, especially when you're exhausted, overworked, and out of rhythm. It reframes habit, not as mindless repetition, but as intentional rehearsal. And it reminds us that resilience doesn't begin with motivation. It begins with what we practice in the dark.

In the quiet space between two shifts, there's a moment where you face something more daunting than your biology: yourself. Not the science, but the silence. The moment when knowledge collides with inertia. You've read the research. You understand the risks. You've even underlined the parts of this book that felt urgent. And yet you still find yourself skipping the cold shower, grabbing the food you swore you'd avoid, or scrolling under fluorescent light at 3:47 a.m. with a brain that knows better. This is not failure. This is the gap between knowing and becoming.

Long before circadian rhythms were studied, before cortisol curves and melatonin pulses were measured, Aristotle gave us a truth that neuroscience is only beginning to reclaim: "We are what we repeatedly do. Excellence, then, is not an act, but a habit." This wasn't motivational fluff. It was the foundation of virtue ethics, the belief that repeated action becomes identity, that practice forges character. In modern terms, practice rewires identity.

You don't become consistent by deciding once. You become consistent by doing, over and over, until your nervous system prefers the new version of you. Aristotle didn't divide people into good or bad, only practiced or unpracticed. Which means the question isn't "Why haven't I changed?" It's "What am I rehearsing?"

Modern neuroscience, however, has largely reduced habit to something unconscious, a neurological shortcut, an automation of behavior rooted in the basal ganglia. This version, inspired by William James, sees habit as mental efficiency: reflexive, thoughtless, automatic. James considered habits a way to offload cognition, to conserve mental effort.[73] This "habit-as-routine" lens emphasizes neural grooves and energy conservation. And while useful, it leaves little room for growth, intention, or transformation. If habits are merely unconscious, then they tell us nothing about how we evolve, or how we move from fatigue to resilience.

Aristotle offers a richer model, what we might call "habit-as-learning." In his view, habit (hexis) is not mindless repetition, but embodied knowledge: a disposition formed through intentional practice. He categorized habits into three domains.[68] Theoretical habits—*knowing that something is true*—are the bedrock of understanding and principle. Behavioral habits—*knowing how to behave*—train reason to govern emotion, to do the right thing until doing the right thing becomes who you are. And technical habits—*knowing how to do*—are skills honed by deliberate repetition, whether suturing, writing, or solving problems. In this view, habits are not what bypass thought, they are what encode it. Not barriers to growth, but the very engine of transformation.

These reframing mindsets change everything for the shift worker. Because if habits are mechanical, your job is to replace one unconscious pattern with another. But if habits are cognitive and identity-driven, then each repetition becomes a conscious rehearsal for who you're becoming. You're not simply trying to "sleep more" or "cut caffeine." You're becoming someone who protects their rhythm. That's not about a decision—it's about a practice. And practices require starting. You don't wait to feel motivated. You start tired, distracted, or imperfect. You fake it, then repeat it, until it's no longer fake. That's not pretending. That's neuroplasticity.

If you want to build new rhythms, don't chase intensity, chase identity. Let it start with something laughably small. Sit in silence for sixty seconds before bed. Leave your walking shoes by the door after your shift. Hook your blackout curtain before you head out the door. Lay out your magnesium. Open your sleep log and write just one sentence. These are not hacks. They are declarations. Not of effort, but of identity. Repeated often enough, they no longer need to be forced. They become part of who you are.

And you won't get there alone. The science is clear: habits that are visible are more likely to stick. Social exposure becomes scaffolding for your new identity. It's why runners post their mileage. Why 12-step programs rely on community. You're not just showing up for yourself. You're showing up for the version of yourself you declared in front of someone else. Repetition witnessed becomes commitment. And commitment is harder to abandon than good intentions.

Let's also be honest: knowing doesn't always feel good. Sometimes, knowledge makes the weight heavier.

Shift Work and Female Rhythm Disruption

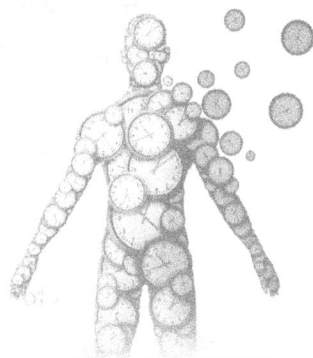

Shift work doesn't affect everyone the same way. In my years as a nurse, I've seen its deepest toll in women—physiological, hormonal, emotional. That makes this chapter more than biology. It makes it personal, for me as a witness, and for many of you as lived experience.

From an evolutionary and physiological standpoint, the female body is governed by two foundational imperatives: survival and reproduction. In that order.

And when the body perceives threat—whether through sleep deprivation, circadian disruption, or chronic stress—it does what it was designed to do: it protects the first by downregulating the second.

This isn't a flaw. It's biology.

Under the strain of shift work, female physiology responds differently than male physiology. It adapts, but at a cost: weight gain, menstrual irregularity, increased risk for polycystic ovarian syndrome (PCOS), and fertility challenges.

These aren't flaws—they're biological alarms. The body's attempt to survive in an environment it was never built for.

This chapter unpacks that response, not to alarm you, but to equip you with the science and strategies your biology has been waiting for.

With knowledge.

With context.

And with tools that may help you reclaim a rhythm that shift work tries to take away.

Shift work doesn't just disrupt your schedule, it rewires your hormonal axis. Before the science of sleep, there was the silence of burnout. This chapter opens where most conversations end: in the space between knowing what's true, and living like it.

Female fertility is a symphony of biological timing. It is a breathtakingly precise orchestration of hormonal rhythms, all cycling in harmony with the body's master circadian clock.[74] For millions of women working night shifts or rotating schedules, however, this symphony is thrown into chaos. Hormonal cascades that are meant to align with sunlight and sleep are blunted, shifted, or silenced, disrupting ovulation, menstrual regularity, and long-term reproductive health.[75]

The female reproductive system is uniquely governed by two interconnected clocks: the daily 24-hour circadian rhythm and the roughly 28-day menstrual cycle. These two systems are in constant communication. Hormonal fluctuations throughout the menstrual cycle affect circadian processes like core body temperature and sleep architecture.[76]

For example, during the luteal phase (the second half of the cycle), core body temperature rises and the rhythm of key hormones like melatonin and cortisol can be dampened.[77] In turn, a stable circadian rhythm, driven by the master clock in the SCN, is essential for regulating the release of reproductive hormones like estradiol, progesterone, and luteinizing hormone (LH).[78] When circadian rhythm is disrupted by shift work, this delicate hormonal balance is destabilized, increasing the risk for irregular cycles and impaired fertility.[74]

At the center of this disruption is melatonin. More than just a sleep hormone, melatonin is a key guardian of reproductive function.[79] Secreted by the brain in response to darkness, it helps regulate the hormonal signals from the brain to the ovaries (the HPO axis), provides crucial antioxidant protection to the developing egg, and even helps promote uterine contractions to time labor, which naturally tends to occur at night.[80] When a woman is exposed to bright light during her biological night, melatonin production is suppressed. This single act can interfere with ovulation, impair fertility, and disrupt the natural timing of birth.[81]

The evidence of this disruption is no longer theoretical; it is documented in large-scale human studies. Research covering over 120,000 women has established an undeniable link between shift work and reproductive dysfunction.[82] Female shift workers report a significantly higher incidence of irregular or prolonged menstrual cycles.[83] Those on rotating shifts face an 80% increase in the risk of infertility and a 30% greater risk of early spontaneous pregnancy loss.[83] Time to conception is longer, and the need for assisted reproductive technologies is higher.[82,83] Even when pregnancy is achieved, shift work is associated with elevated risks for both preterm labor and post-term birth.[84]

The damage extends across a woman's entire reproductive lifespan. A 22-year study of U.S. nurses found that long-term rotating shift work was associated with a 22% increased risk of early menopause (before age 45).[85] This is not a trivial outcome, as early menopause carries with it increased risks for cardiovascular disease, osteoporosis, and reduced life expectancy.[86]

Understanding this deep biological conflict isn't just a personal concern—it's a public health imperative. As more women enter professions that demand around-the-clock coverage, we must confront the physiological trade-offs baked into the system.

Circadian disruption doesn't just affect sleep or metabolism, it reverberates through the hormonal axis, impacting ovulation, fertility, and long-term reproductive health.

But knowledge is power.

By grounding healthcare decisions in the science of chronobiology, we can equip female shift workers with tools to protect their reproductive health, not just in the short term, but across the full span of their careers and lives.

Clock Notes

Circadian-Menstrual Coupling – The interaction between the body's 24-hour circadian rhythm and the 28-day menstrual cycle, which co-regulate hormonal release, sleep patterns, and reproductive timing.

Melatonin Suppression – The reduction of melatonin production due to nighttime light exposure, which can impair ovulation, disrupt the HPO axis, and alter the timing of labor.

HPO Axis (Hypothalamic-Pituitary-Ovarian Axis) – The hormonal signaling pathway that coordinates reproductive function; highly sensitive to circadian rhythm disruption from shift work.

Luteal Phase Disruption – Alterations in the second half of the menstrual cycle where progesterone and temperature rhythms are especially vulnerable to circadian misalignment.

Early Menopause Risk – The increased likelihood of menopause occurring before age 45 among long-term rotating shift workers, with associated risks for cardiovascular disease and reduced longevity.

How Shift Work Breaks Male Hormonal Rhythms

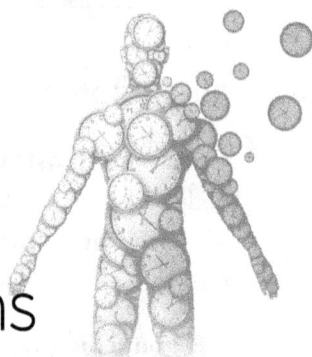

For men, testosterone is the hormonal driver of strength, energy, and sexual health.[87] But it doesn't run on demand, it runs on rhythm. Every 24 hours, testosterone follows a powerful circadian cycle, peaking in the morning to prepare the body for the demands of the day.[87]

But for the man working against the clock, that rhythm doesn't rise; it collapses. The rotating shifts, long nights, and erratic schedules of shift work fracture this natural cycle, disrupting the male endocrine system and unraveling energy, libido, and fertility.[87]

While the effects of shift work on female hormones are well-documented, its impact on the male hormonal cascade, particularly on testosterone and its precursor, pregnenolone, has long been underexplored.

But that gap is finally starting to close. And the findings are sobering. A recent study of male shift workers with shift work sleep disorder found a striking pattern: significantly reduced levels of testosterone and pregnenolone compared to their non-shift-working counterparts.[88]

I've worked alongside men whose strength seemed untouchable. But years of overnight shifts told a different story: tired eyes, foggy mornings, relationships strained under the weight of exhaustion they couldn't explain.

But the damage didn't stop there. It is part of a larger, systemic breakdown. The same study found that these men were not only hormonally compromised but also metabolically stressed. They tended to have a higher Body Mass Index (BMI) and a greater prevalence of hypertension, diabetes, and high cholesterol.[89]

This is the direct result of a lifestyle dictated by circadian disruption—irregular meals, late-night eating, and poor sleep—which destabilizes the body's ability to manage metabolism and intersects directly with reproductive health.

The damage extends into the most intimate aspects of a man's health. Researchers now believe there is a direct pathway linking shift work to conditions like premature ejaculation (PE).[90]

Men with SWSD report higher levels of anxiety and depression, states known to affect key neurotransmitters like serotonin and dopamine.[91] These same neurotransmitters are essential for both sleep regulation and sexual function. When they become dysregulated, the risk of PE, compromised erectile function, and hypogonadism (low testosterone) increases.[92]

The final consequence is perhaps the most personal: fertility. In a study of men undergoing fertility evaluation, those working night or rotating shifts exhibited significantly poorer semen quality.[93] They were more likely to have a low sperm count (oligozoospermia) and a lower percentage of normally shaped sperm.[93] The study revealed a direct link between sleep and fertility: total sleep duration was positively correlated with sperm concentration, and the time it took to fall asleep was linked to a lower total sperm count.[94] Crucially, even after accounting for other factors like age and stress, the circadian misalignment of shift work remained a powerful, independent predictor of reduced sperm quality.

The evidence is no longer theoretical. A life lived against the clock is not just exhausting, it's erosive. To testosterone. To resilience. To reproductive health itself.

Clock Notes

Testosterone Rhythm Disruption – A shift in the natural peak of testosterone production, typically highest in the morning, caused by night shifts and irregular schedules, leading to fatigue, low libido, and mood changes.

Pregnenolone Decline – A reduction in the precursor hormone to testosterone, observed in male shift workers, contributing to broader endocrine dysfunction and reduced vitality.

Circadian-Linked Sexual Dysfunction – The disruption of serotonin and dopamine pathways by shift work, impairing sexual function and increasing risk of premature ejaculation and erectile dysfunction.

Sperm Quality Decline – Reduced semen quality, including low sperm count and abnormal morphology, linked to sleep deprivation and circadian misalignment in male shift workers.

Compromised Vascular Infrastructure

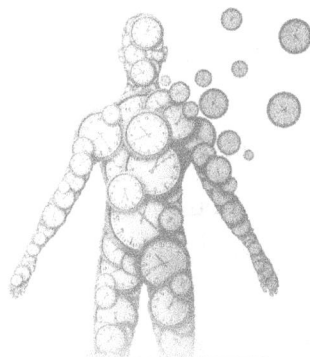

With every flipped schedule and fluorescent-lit night, the damage of shift work goes deeper than fatigue. It strikes the very scaffolding of our biology: the vast, intricate network of arteries and veins that deliver life to every cell.

This isn't just plumbing. It's a timed, intelligent infrastructure, one that pulses with rhythm. It runs on a clock, its own precise circadian rhythm. And when that clock is broken, the system doesn't just slow down; it begins to erode from within.

For shift workers, cardiovascular disease doesn't begin in the heart—it begins in time. It is an upstream catastrophe triggered by a lifestyle lived against the clock, where disrupted sleep and misaligned meals unleash a cascade of chronic harm.[95]

Epidemiological data now identify shift work as a significant, independent risk factor for a host of cardiovascular diseases, including hypertension, coronary artery disease, and sudden cardiac death.[96]

The mechanism? A perfect storm of circadian disruption. Clock misalignment destabilizes vascular homeostasis, sending the autonomic nervous system into chronic overdrive, raising blood pressure and distorting lipid metabolism.[95]

Second, this misalignment activates systemic inflammation. Shift workers consistently show higher levels of inflammatory markers like C-reactive protein (CRP) and interleukin-6, which promote endothelial dysfunction, a condition where the lining of the blood vessels becomes damaged and less flexible.[97]

Together, inflammation and oxidative stress drive atherosclerosis, the slow hardening and clogging of the arteries.[98]

Interestingly, our vascular tissues are remarkably resilient. Unlike the liver and pancreas, which react quickly to circadian disruption, the aorta resists longer, making vascular damage a late but deadly consequence of chronic stress.[99] This suggests that vascular damage requires the kind of prolonged, compounded stress that is the hallmark of a career in shift work. Over time, this chronic assault overwhelms the system.

The core clock genes—CLOCK, BMAL1, and PER2—aren't just timekeepers. They play a direct role in maintaining the health and function of your blood vessels. These genes help regulate the delicate balance of blood clotting, arterial dilation, and vascular tone, the factors that keep blood flowing smoothly and prevent catastrophic events like heart attacks and strokes.

When these genes are disrupted, the vascular scaffolding begins to fail, creating an upstream cause of the systemic metabolic dysfunction that contributes to obesity and diabetes.[100]

Finally, shift work traps the body in a state of chronic, low-grade emergency. The "fight-or-flight" response, designed to be a short-term survival mechanism, becomes the new baseline.

Stress hormones like catecholamines remain elevated, flooding the system hour after hour. [101] Blood pressure rises. Cholesterol and glucose levels skew. The body stays locked in a state of metabolic readiness that never fully resolves.

This isn't stress. It's erosion. It's a slow, physiological burn, one that wears down systems built for recovery, not permanence.

This combination of sympathetic overdrive, metabolic chaos, and chronic inflammation creates the ideal conditions for vascular injury, accelerating the path toward cardiovascular disease.[102]

Clock Notes

Vascular Circadian Rhythm - The intrinsic biological timing system within the cardiovascular system that governs blood pressure, vessel tone, and clotting patterns; disrupted by shift work and poor sleep.

Endothelial Dysfunction - Impairment of the inner lining of blood vessels, often triggered by inflammation and oxidative stress, leading to poor vascular flexibility and increased risk of atherosclerosis.

Atherosclerosis - The gradual buildup of plaques in the arterial walls, accelerated by chronic inflammation and circadian misalignment common in long-term shift workers.

Sympathetic Overdrive - A chronic activation of the body's stress response system, marked by elevated catecholamines and sustained high blood pressure, which strains the cardiovascular system over time.

When the Heart Falls Out Of Time

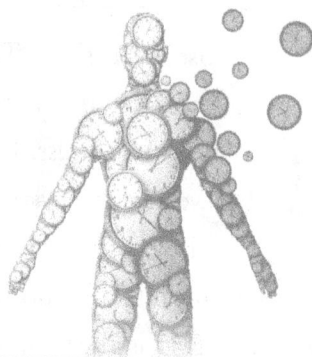

We call the heart the engine of life, but an engine alone cannot move—without its chassis, it has nowhere to go.

Your arteries, veins, and capillaries form more than a circulatory map—they are the roads themselves. They're a living framework, responsive, rhythmic, and exquisitely timed to the demands of day and night. Blood flow isn't static. It pulses with intention, adapting to sleep, activity, light, food, and stress.

But when shift work distorts the schedule, the vascular system doesn't rebel. It adapts—quietly, chronically, and at a cost.

It narrows. It stiffens. It forgets how to relax.

Over time, this network loses its responsiveness. Not just in the heart, but in the brain, kidneys, extremities, and every organ that relies on oxygen and nutrient delivery.

This chapter isn't just about heart attacks or strokes. It's about the slow degradation of a system designed to move with the rhythm of life.

Because when the vascular system falls out of time, nothing—nothing—functions as it should.

So here's your moment of pause: If your vessels are the highways of your life, how many detours have you forced them to take? And how long can they keep rerouting before they fail to deliver you where you need to go?

But vascular damage is just the beginning. The clock's misalignment culminates where timing matters most: the heart.

For the shift worker, the most dangerous part of the day is often the dawn. This isn't theoretical, it's a measurable, slow-motion catastrophe triggered by the body's internal clock. These chaotic schedules fracture the body's natural cycle long before the first symptom appears. A silent strain is building inside the cardiovascular system.

With every disrupted night, the delicate, life-sustaining rhythms that protect the heart begin to fray. Inflammation rises. Arteries stiffen. A cascade of vascular damage begins to unfold.

The link between our circadian rhythm and our heart is undeniable. One of the most powerful illustrations of this connection comes from a landmark study that tracked the timing of nearly 3,000 heart attacks. The pattern was stark and unambiguous: heart attacks occurred three times more often in the early morning than in the late evening, with a clear peak around 9 a.m.[103] This morning surge is not unique to heart attacks. Subsequent, larger analyses have shown that stroke, dangerous arrhythmias, and aortic dissection all follow the same predictable daily rhythm.[104] The timing doesn't just affect frequency; it affects severity. Heart attacks that strike in the morning are consistently larger and have worse clinical outcomes.[103]

What drives this deadly morning vulnerability? It's a convergence of our natural rhythms. Upon waking, a surge of cortisol and an activation of the sympathetic nervous system create a pro-thrombotic, or clot-promoting, environment.[105] For a healthy person, this is a normal part of the daily cycle. For the shift worker, whose body is already under the chronic stress of circadian misalignment, this daily peak becomes a window of extreme risk.

Tools like carotid ultrasound and high-sensitivity CRP now reveal this damage long before symptoms appear.

Studies using carotid artery ultrasounds show that years of shift work are directly correlated with an increased thickness of the artery walls (carotid intima-media thickness) and elevated CRP, both clear markers of atherosclerosis and systemic inflammation.[106] This is the silent progression of cardiovascular disease, visible even in young and otherwise healthy individuals.

This is where the intersection of lifestyle and biology becomes critical. In studies examining these vascular changes, one factor emerged as a powerful buffer against the strain: physical activity. Participants who maintained a routine of high-intensity aerobic exercise showed measurable improvements in vascular health, including lower arterial stiffness.[107] This aligns with a broader body of evidence showing that intense exercise doesn't just build endurance; it dampens inflammation, promotes the healthy dilation of blood vessels, and helps preserve the integrity of our vascular system in the face of circadian disruption.[108]

Even brief sessions of high-intensity training, performed just three times a week, have been shown to lower blood pressure and improve cholesterol profiles.[109]

This research signals a necessary shift in how we approach cardiovascular prevention.

The damage doesn't begin with a diagnosis. It begins earlier—quietly, incrementally—unfolding over years of circadian disruption. Traditional screenings often miss the warning signs.

Shift workers can present with normal blood pressure and cholesterol levels, even as silent inflammation and vascular strain accumulate beneath the surface.

To address the true burden of shift work, we must move beyond static snapshots of health. That means integrating circadian-aware diagnostics, like high-sensitivity CRP, and recognizing early-stage dysfunction before it becomes irreversible.

Prevention starts not with symptoms, but with timing.

Clock Notes

Morning Cardiovascular Vulnerability - A circadian-driven surge in cardiovascular events, particularly heart attacks and strokes, peaking around 9 a.m. due to hormonal and sympathetic nervous system activation.

Carotid Intima-Media Thickness (CIMT) - A diagnostic marker for atherosclerosis; increased CIMT is associated with long-term shift work and indicates early vascular damage.

C-Reactive Protein (CRP) - A sensitive inflammatory biomarker elevated in shift workers, used to detect subclinical cardiovascular strain before overt symptoms develop.

Pro-Thrombotic State - A clot-promoting physiological condition triggered by the circadian cortisol surge upon waking, increasing risk for acute cardiac events in misaligned individuals.

How Fat Turns Against Us

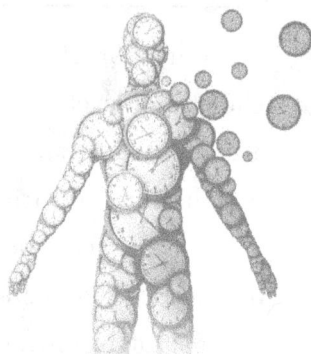

For decades, body fat was seen as little more than insulation, an inert storage depot for excess calories. But that view is outdated. And dangerously incomplete. We now know that fat is anything but passive.

Fat is dynamic, endocrine, and highly time-sensitive.

It secretes hormones through a constant stream of chemical messengers called adipokines. Your white adipose tissue (WAT) is in constant conversation with the rest of your body, influencing everything from hunger and immunity to inflammation and blood sugar control.[110]

In a healthy, synchronized system, this tissue is a masterful keeper of metabolic balance. But when you work against the clock, the rhythm inside your fat cells unravels. What was once an organ of survival becomes a primary source of chronic, low-grade inflammation. For the shift worker, obesity-associated metabolic stress triggers a profound shift in the WAT, causing it to secrete pro-inflammatory adipokines that drive systemic dysfunction and contribute directly to the development of type 2 diabetes.[111]

This is a direct consequence of the body's peripheral clocks losing their way, a process that impairs the fundamental function of our fat tissue. The body's other fat, brown adipose tissue (BAT), also falls victim to this disruption. Long recognized as a thermogenic, or heat-producing, organ, BAT is now understood to be a critical regulator of our overall metabolic rate.[112]

But when the circadian rhythm is broken, BAT's metabolic fire is dampened. Its ability to burn energy efficiently is compromised, making it harder to maintain a healthy weight.[113]

At the heart of this dysfunction are the core clock genes, particularly BMAL1. This single gene has demonstrated a profound influence on lipid metabolism and the health of our fat cells.[114]

In experimental models where BMAL1 is suppressed in fat tissue, researchers observe enlarged fat cells, even in the absence of inflammation.[110] This reveals that circadian disruption can damage metabolism independent of overt obesity or inflammation.[115] This stunning finding suggests that circadian disruption can damage our metabolic health through multiple pathways, attacking the very structure and function of our fat cells independent of other factors.[116]

Adipose tissue was never passive—it's a rhythmic communicator. When that rhythm fractures, its protective loyalty turns into chronic sabotage. What once protected you starts working against you, slowly, quietly, and dangerously.

White and brown fat are not static repositories of energy. They are dynamic, anticipatory organs, sensitive to light, food, temperature, hormones, and most of all, time. Like every other major system in the body, adipose tissue is governed by a circadian blueprint, a set of molecular rhythms that align its function with the 24-hour cycle of life. When that blueprint is ignored, altered, or overwritten, as it often is in the world of shift work, the consequences become metabolic and cardiovascular liabilities.

That's not an abstract warning. It's a biological sequence. When you eat at night, particularly high-glycemic, quickly digested carbohydrates, your white adipose tissue responds sluggishly. Why? Because it was never designed to handle glucose during your biological night.

Mild insulin resistance in adipose tissue during nighttime hours is not a flaw; it's an evolutionary feature, a protective mechanism to conserve glucose for the brain. But in the modern shift work environment, where eating windows are often misaligned with internal clocks, that adaptive feature becomes a metabolic trap.

The damage doesn't stop there. Circadian disruption also blunts insulin secretion from the pancreas.[117] So now, not only is your fat tissue less responsive to insulin, but there's less insulin to go around. The result? Blood glucose spikes, metabolic inflexibility, and elevated long-term risk for insulin resistance and type 2 diabetes.[112] Add in reduced physical activity, disrupted sleep, and irregular eating patterns, and the stage is set for cardiometabolic collapse—one snack, one soda, one night shift at a time.

But here's the paradox: the same system that creates vulnerability also reveals a path toward resilience. Time-restricted eating, particularly during the biological day, has emerged as a powerful intervention to restore rhythm, reduce glucose variability, and stabilize insulin response, even in simulated shift work environments.[118] Strategic alignment of meals with your internal clock, eating when your biology expects it, can buffer some of the worst metabolic consequences of working against nature.

And yet, even that isn't a cure-all. Shift work imposes multifactorial risk—genetic, behavioral, environmental, and institutional. That's why the path forward isn't one-size-fits-all. It requires a personalized, multidisciplinary approach—one that includes not just meal timing, but light exposure, sleep optimization, metabolic tracking, and adaptive protocols that respond to the realities of 24/7 life.

Adipose tissue doesn't just store calories. It keeps score. And what it's tracking isn't just how much you eat, but *when* you eat, *how* you sleep, and *whether your rhythms are aligned or ignored.*

The shift worker doesn't just need another diet plan.

They need a clock-aware metabolism strategy, one that recognizes fat as both a partner and a risk, and that uses time itself as a therapeutic tool.

The conclusion is unavoidable: The circadian clock within the adipocyte is essential to the health of both white and brown fat.[119] When shift work throws that clock into disarray, the consequences ripple outward.

Metabolic flexibility declines. Energy balance falters.

And the very organ designed to protect us in times of scarcity becomes a driver of chronic disease. What was once a survival mechanism now fuels our slow undoing.

Clock Notes

Adipokines – Chemical messengers secreted by fat cells that regulate hunger, immunity, inflammation, and glucose metabolism, disrupted by circadian misalignment.

White Adipose Tissue (WAT) – A hormonally active fat storage organ that, under shift-induced circadian disruption, secretes pro-inflammatory signals contributing to metabolic disease.

Brown Adipose Tissue (BAT) – A heat-producing fat tissue that regulates metabolic rate; its energy-burning capacity is suppressed when circadian rhythms are misaligned.

BMAL1 – A core circadian gene that controls lipid metabolism and fat cell function; its disruption alters fat storage patterns and impairs adipose tissue health.

Metabolic Flexibility – The body's ability to switch between burning fat and glucose; compromised when circadian-regulated fat cell activity is impaired.

The Silent Organ Shift

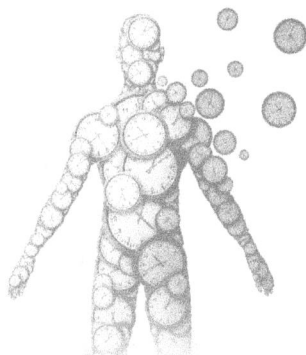

The liver and pancreas are the tireless frontline workers of metabolism. They clock in early, respond without delay, and never miss a shift, until the rhythms that guide them begin to break.

They do more than process fuel—they are masterful timekeepers, working in a tightly coordinated rhythm to manage blood sugar, store energy, detoxify the body, and regulate fat metabolism.[120]

This precision is governed by their own internal circadian clocks, which are meant to be in lockstep with the brain's master clock. But when shift work flips the daily cycle, it throws these vital organs into a state of chronic, damaging chaos. The silent shift of the clock becomes a silent assault from within.

The damage is not abstract. For the shift worker, it manifests as creeping weight gain, elevated liver enzymes, and the first signs of insulin resistance. Research has now drawn a direct line between night shift work and the progression of non-alcoholic fatty liver disease (NAFLD), where the liver's metabolic function is so impaired it accumulates excessive fat.[121] This condition, exacerbated by the hormonal and dietary realities of a life lived against the clock, can escalate to non-alcoholic steatohepatitis (NASH) and even heighten the risk of liver cancer.[122] The link is so strong that elevated liver enzymes have become a reliable marker for the metabolic dysfunction caused by circadian disruption.[123]

The pancreas is the other frontline casualty. Its -cells, which are responsible for producing and secreting insulin, also possess their own autonomous circadian clocks.

Insulin release is not meant to be constant; it follows a daily rhythm designed to align with our feeding and fasting cycles. In metabolic dysfunction, clock genes PER2, PER3, and CRY2 become blunted, disrupting insulin release precisely when it matters most.[124]

This genetic evidence provides a direct link between a broken clock and the failure of the pancreas to release insulin effectively.[125] These clock genes are the master regulators of our 24-hour cycle. PER2 is central to maintaining the rhythm and supporting glucose metabolism, while CRY2 helps stabilize the entire system and is crucial for regulating insulin secretion.[126]

Environmental factors—like high-fat diets, misaligned eating windows, and fragmented sleep—pour fuel on the fire, further disrupting the expression of these genes within the pancreas and accelerating the path to β-cell failure.[127]

The evidence from clock gene studies is perhaps the most compelling. In mice with BMAL1 knocked out in pancreatic tissue, researchers observe high blood glucose and insulin resistance, even without a high-fat diet.[128]

This doesn't happen because the pancreas can't produce insulin.

It happens because it can't produce it *on time*. The pancreatic clock has lost its rhythm, and with it, the ability to maintain metabolic balance. This research underscores a critical truth: the liver and pancreas are not passive casualties of poor diet or disrupted sleep. They are active, time-keeping organs, finely tuned to the body's internal clocks. And shift work wages a direct war on that biology.

Clock Notes

Non-Alcoholic Fatty Liver Disease (NAFLD) – A metabolic liver condition marked by excess fat accumulation, strongly linked to circadian disruption from night shift work.

PER2 / PER3 / CRY2 – Clock genes involved in regulating insulin secretion and glucose metabolism; their downregulation in shift workers contributes to -cell dysfunction.

Liver Enzymes – Biomarkers such as ALT and AST that rise in response to liver stress; commonly elevated in shift workers experiencing metabolic strain.

Pancreatic Clock – An internal circadian system within the pancreas that controls insulin release in alignment with feeding cycles; disrupted by erratic schedules and poor diet.

How Circadian Rhythms Shape Strength

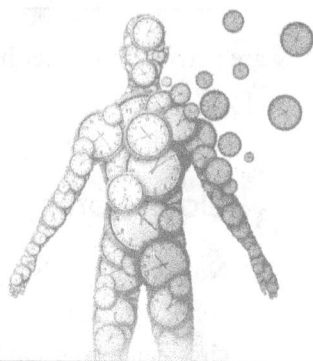

At 3:00 a.m., a nurse grabs vending machine snacks between call bells. Her legs ache. Her posture slumps. And inside her muscle cells, a clock is ticking—out of time.

Skeletal muscle is your metabolic shield, and in the shift worker, that shield is constantly under siege. It stores strength, buffers fatigue, and regulates whole-body health. But disrupted sleep, stress, and mistimed meals turn this vital tissue into a site of silent decline.

Far from passive tissue, muscle is constantly in motion, rebuilding, repairing, and responding to an intricate symphony of signals from sleep, stress, and nutrition.

Shift work dulls the body's natural anabolic (muscle-building) signals, disrupts protein synthesis, and throws hormonal balance into disarray.[129]

Like every other tissue we've explored, muscle operates on a strict internal schedule, governed by core clock genes like CLOCK and BMAL1.[130] When these genes are disrupted, the consequences are immediate and severe. Animal studies show that muscle-specific deletion of BMAL1 leads directly to muscle atrophy, weakness, and impaired glucose uptake, even without any changes in diet or physical activity.[131]

This damage is amplified by sleep loss. Under normal conditions, our muscles are in a constant, balanced state of breakdown and repair. But numerous studies have shown that even a single night of total sleep deprivation is enough to reduce muscle protein synthesis, increase protein breakdown, and disrupt the expression of clock genes in human muscle tissue.[132]

In one study, calorie-restricted individuals who were sleep-deprived lost 60% more muscle mass than their well-rested counterparts on the exact same diet.[133]

Sleep loss also dysregulates appetite hormones, leading to cravings for the high-carbohydrate, low-protein foods that are least effective for muscle repair.[134]

This isn't just about losing strength, it's about losing resilience in the very tissue that protects against diabetes, weight gain, and accelerated aging.[129]

So, how can a shift worker fight back? The research points to two powerful, synergistic strategies: strategic protein intake and resistance training. Skeletal muscle stores up to 75% of the body's protein, and it requires a steady supply to maintain itself, especially during periods of stress and circadian misalignment.[135]

Evidence suggests that distributing an intake of 20–30 grams of high-quality protein across several meals is the most effective way to maximize muscle protein synthesis.[136]

For the shift worker, this means aligning protein intake with your internal clock, not just external time cues. A strategic, protein-rich meal during an overnight shift can be a powerful tool to offset muscle breakdown.[137]

The other key is resistance training, one of the most potent stimulators of muscle growth. While fatigue can make exercise feel impossible, even short, intense sessions can defend against insulin resistance and protect muscle mass.[138]

Overcoming the motivation gap is critical. Studies on the "Köhler effect" show that training with a partner, even a virtual partner, can significantly increase effort and consistency during workouts.[139]

For the shift worker, muscle is more than a source of strength—it's a metabolic shield. Protecting it is essential for defending against insulin resistance, unwanted weight gain, and long-term metabolic decline.

Because in the world of circadian disruption, strength isn't just physical—it's your most powerful survival strategy.

Clock Notes

Muscle Protein Synthesis – The process of building new muscle proteins, highly sensitive to sleep, feeding patterns, and circadian signals; suppressed by shift work and sleep deprivation.

Köhler Effect – A motivational phenomenon where training alongside a partner enhances workout effort and intensity, useful for combating shift-related fatigue and maintaining exercise adherence.

Strategic Protein Intake – The practice of distributing 20–30g of high-quality protein across waking hours to support muscle maintenance and synthesis, especially critical for shift workers during overnight periods.

The Fast-Forward Button on the Brain

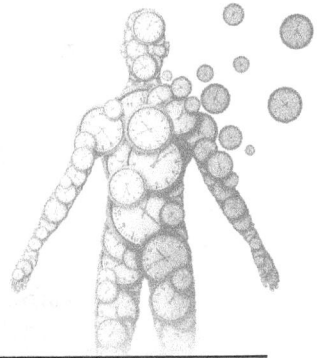

The damage of shift work doesn't stop at the physical, it reaches deep into the brain. Shift work doesn't just tax the body, it rewires the brain. Nights and rotating shifts alter the structure and function of your neural circuits.

For every nurse, paramedic, and overnight factory worker who has felt their focus slip or their memory falter—you're not imagining it. The neuroscience has caught up. A life lived against the clock doesn't just strain the mind. It can accelerate brain aging.

The brain runs on exquisite timing.

Its master clock, tucked within the hypothalamus, governs far more than sleep: it shapes memory, attention, emotional regulation, and even the pace of neurological recovery.[140]

But shift work scrambles these essential signals. And over time, that disruption doesn't just fade, it layers, accumulates, and amplifies.

Emerging research now confirms what many have long suspected: the neurological impact of circadian misalignment can be long-lasting, lingering for years even after returning to a regular schedule.[141]

In one study, biological models exposed to rotating shift work experienced worse stroke outcomes, delayed recovery, and higher mortality rates, effects that remained long after the disruptive schedule ended.[142]

The findings were particularly concerning for female subjects, who experienced more severe deficits. The pattern mirrors the real-world demographics of shift work, where women make up the majority of overnight healthcare and caregiving roles.

To quantify this "aging" effect, scientists have developed a powerful biomarker called the Brain Age Index (BAI). Derived from sleep EEG data, a higher BAI suggests that a person's brain is aging faster than their chronological years would predict.[143] Recent studies have delivered a sobering verdict: night-shift workers consistently show higher BAI values than their day-working peers.[143] The longer an individual works nights, the greater the impact, with poor-quality daytime sleep and a reduction in deep, restorative sleep being the primary drivers of this accelerated aging.[142]

This is not an abstract finding. It has real-world consequences. Firefighters with poor sleep quality show reduced volume in the hippocampus, a brain region critical for memory and emotional regulation.[144] Slower executive functions, like decision-making, are all well-documented cognitive impairments common among shift workers.[145]

Yet there is a paradox within the data that offers a lifeline. While many shift workers show these clear structural and functional brain changes, others show little to no measurable damage. Why? The answer appears to be the quality of their sleep. Across studies, the neurological deficits were most pronounced in workers who struggled with sleep, those with disrupted REM, poor deep sleep, and frequent awakenings.[146]

This suggests that it's not just the timing of the shift that matters, it's the quality of the recovery sleep that may be the most critical factor. The science is sobering: shift work can accelerate brain aging. But it also points to our most powerful line of defense.

Clock Notes

Brain Age Index (BAI) – A biomarker derived from sleep EEG data that estimates the biological age of the brain; consistently elevated in night shift workers, indicating accelerated neurological aging.

Hippocampal Atrophy – Shrinkage of the brain's memory and emotion-regulation center, observed in sleep-deprived shift workers, contributing to cognitive decline and mood dysregulation.

REM and Deep Sleep Disruption – A hallmark of shift work-related neurological decline; poor-quality restorative sleep is the key driver of cognitive impairment, even more than shift timing alone.

Neurological Resilience – The observed ability of some shift workers to avoid cognitive decline, strongly associated with maintaining high-quality sleep despite circadian disruption.

Cancer and the Clock

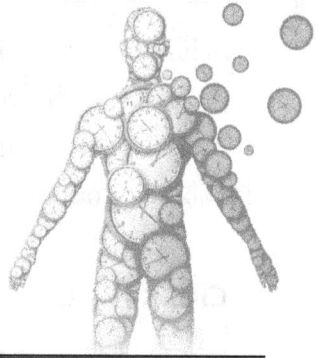

Cancer is a heavy word. We tend to think of it in terms of heredity, chemical exposure, or radiation. But for shift workers, the risk runs deeper, rooted in a broken biological clock.

It's not just an occupational hazard, already identified as a probable carcinogen. It's a biological collision.

Your circadian system doesn't just regulate sleep. It governs the timing of DNA repair, immune surveillance, and cell cycle checkpoints, the body's internal safeguards against malignancy.[147]

When those rhythms unravel, so does your defense.

Emerging research confirms what many suspected: disruption of circadian timing promotes genomic instability and accelerates cancer risk.[147]

Core clock genes like BMAL1 and CLOCK, once guardians of cellular order, can be hijacked, activating tumor-promoting pathways, silencing tumor suppressors like p53 and creating the perfect storm for disease to take hold.[148,149]

These genes normally regulate the most critical anti-cancer processes: cell cycle control, genomic stability, and apoptosis. When that regulation breaks down, the body's defenses collapse from within.[150]

This internal timing system doesn't just influence cancer risk; it also dramatically affects the efficacy and toxicity of cancer treatments.[151] This has given rise to a groundbreaking field called chronotherapy, which seeks to time treatments to the body's natural rhythms.

Chronobiology isn't just a framework for prevention—it may be the future of precision treatment. And for shift workers, timing could be the most powerful therapy they never knew they needed.

The enzymes that metabolize chemotherapy drugs and the cellular machinery that repairs DNA all operate on a strict circadian schedule.[151] By administering chemotherapy or radiation when cancer cells are most vulnerable and healthy cells are most resilient, oncologists can significantly improve therapeutic outcomes and reduce devastating side effects.[152]

For example, the metabolism of the common chemotherapy drug 5-fluorouracil (5-FU) fluctuates throughout the day, meaning its effectiveness and toxicity change depending on the hour it's given.[153]

Lifestyle factors endemic to shift work accelerate the breakdown of cellular defenses. Chronic exposure to light at night suppresses the production of melatonin, a hormone with powerful anti-cancer properties.[154] Irregular eating patterns disrupt the peripheral clocks in the liver and pancreas, promoting the kind of metabolic dysfunction and inflammation that are known to drive tumor growth.[155] A misaligned clock can even reprogram cancer cells to adopt the infamous "Warburg effect," a state of hyperactive metabolism that allows tumors to grow at a terrifying rate.[156]

Finally, a broken clock cripples the body's own defenses.

The circadian system is a master regulator of the immune system, controlling the activity of natural killer (NK) cells and T-cells that are responsible for hunting down and eliminating tumors.[157]

When circadian signaling breaks down, immune surveillance falters, giving cancer the window it needs to take hold and spread. But understanding this connection opens a powerful new frontier.

Clock Notes

Melatonin Suppression – Chronic light exposure at night diminishes melatonin production, removing a natural anti-cancer defense and weakening cellular protection against tumor development.

Warburg Effect – A metabolic shift seen in many cancers where cells favor glycolysis even in oxygen-rich environments; may be accelerated by circadian disruption and metabolic chaos.

Immune Surveillance Breakdown – Circadian misalignment impairs the activity of natural killer cells and T-cells, reducing the body's ability to detect and eliminate cancer cells.

Circadian Science in Critical Illness

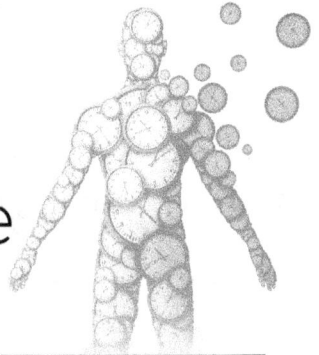

When someone you love is in the intensive care unit (ICU), biology stops being theoretical. It becomes immediate, intimate, and urgent. In the high-stakes world of the ICU, our focus narrows to machines, medications, and interventions. We track vitals, adjust dosages, and fight minute by minute.

But one of the most powerful forces shaping recovery is often overlooked: the rhythm of the patient's own internal clock.

The ICU, by its very nature, is a profoundly anti-circadian environment. The constant artificial light, the unrelenting ambient noise, and the necessity of overnight clinical procedures creates a 24-hour state of emergency that shatters the body's sleep-wake cycle.[158] For a critically ill patient, whose body is already under immense physiological stress, this disruption is catastrophic. It impairs circadian homeostasis and pushes them into a state of metabolic chaos that actively works against healing.[158]

Nowhere is this more evident than in patients with sepsis, a leading cause of ICU admission.[159] This life-threatening response to infection triggers profound mitochondrial dysfunction and endothelial impairment, a breakdown in the core cellular systems responsible for energy production and vascular stability.[159] We now know that the circadian system is a master regulator of these precise cellular processes. When the clock is broken by the ICU environment, it can worsen the organ damage caused by sepsis.

The most visible consequence of this internal chaos is ICU delirium. This state of acute confusion and altered consciousness is not just a temporary side effect; it is a dangerous complication linked to significantly higher rates of long-term cognitive impairment and mortality.[160] At its core lies a breakdown of the sleep-wake cycle, and with it, a flattened secretion of melatonin, the body's master circadian hormone.

But this is where the science offers a powerful glimmer of hope. If a broken clock contributes to the problem, then fixing the clock can be part of the solution. A multicenter randomized controlled trial has already shown that using a melatonin-receptor agonist, ramelteon, can significantly reduce the incidence of ICU delirium.[161]

This finding is part of a paradigm shift in critical care. Building on this evidence, researchers are now proposing a novel, integrated approach to restore circadian rhythms in the most vulnerable patients. This "MEGA bundle" is a series of coordinated, non-pharmacological interventions designed to re-anchor the body's clock. It includes intense light therapy in the morning, cyclic nutritional support that mimics day-night feeding patterns, scheduled physical therapy, and a comprehensive sleep hygiene protocol to minimize light and noise at night.[162]

By aligning the ICU environment with the body's natural rhythms, we can do more than create comfort—we can restore biological coherence. This may improve metabolic regulation, support circadian signaling, and give critically ill patients a better chance to recover, not just survive.

In critical care, the clock is medicine. If you're at the bedside, whether as a clinician or loved one, protect the rhythm: dim the lights at night, reduce noise, and advocate for morning light and scheduled rest. A stable circadian signal may be as life-saving as any drug on the chart.

Clock Notes

ICU Circadian Disruption – The intensive care environment breaks natural light-dark cycles, causing melatonin suppression, sleep-wake disruption, and impaired biological recovery.

ICU Delirium – A serious complication marked by acute confusion and linked to circadian rhythm breakdown and melatonin suppression; strongly associated with worse cognitive and survival outcomes.

Mitochondrial Dysfunction in Sepsis – A hallmark of critical illness where disrupted circadian regulation impairs cellular energy production, compounding organ failure and slowing recovery.

Ramelteon – A melatonin receptor agonist shown to significantly reduce ICU delirium by restoring circadian signaling in critically ill patients.

MEGA Bundle – A comprehensive circadian-alignment strategy in ICU care including bright morning light therapy, rhythmic feeding, scheduled physical activity, and strict nighttime sleep hygiene.

"Give me a place to stand, and a lever long enough, and I will move the world."

— ARCHIMEDES

The Power Laws:
Building Rhythm From
What you Can Control

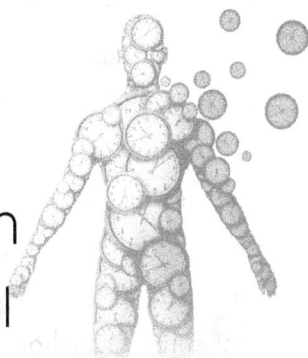

Health isn't the result of a single choice—it's the outcome of a system of choices. And for the shift worker, navigating that system means understanding what I call the Three Power Laws of Health: Sleep, Nutrition, and Exercise.

Not every chapter in this book ends with a clean prescription. Some sections won't offer a silver-bullet solution, because there isn't one.

But there is rhythm. And repetition.

The simple act of repeating when you sleep, when you eat, and when you rise is more powerful than most pills or protocols. These are the most cost-effective tools we possess, anchoring biology in a world designed to pull it apart.

You'll notice these themes repeated often in these pages, and that's intentional. Repetition isn't filler; it's emphasis. Because in truth, rhythm and routine are the strongest levers you have. The science may be complex, but the strategies that matter most are deceptively simple: go to bed at the same time, wake at the same time, eat at the same time. Small patterns, repeated, create stability where shift work erodes it.

Consistency, not complexity, is the lever. A body trained by rhythm will adapt. A body deprived of it will unravel.

When it comes to circadian disruption, metabolic collapse, or cellular burnout, the truth is messier than we'd like. These are not problems with tidy fixes. They're signals, messages from a system under strain. If you're searching for direction—somewhere to begin, something to anchor to, a lever—the answer lies in the Three Power Laws.

All three matter. All three are essential. But in a life lived against the clock, they are not created equal.

Understanding their hierarchy isn't just helpful, it's essential to survival. Sleep is the master pillar, the foundation upon which all other health outcomes rest. It is the single most powerful, non-negotiable biological process we have, governing cellular repair, memory consolidation, and hormonal balance.[163] Yet for the shift worker, it is the most compromised and the least controllable. Fragmented rest and chronic sleep debt aren't flaws—they're features of the job. This deficit doesn't just cause fatigue—it drives the metabolic dysfunction behind obesity, insulin resistance, and type 2 diabetes.[164]

Nutrition is the most emotionally charged, and the most culturally distorted, pillar. It's where cultural habits, personal beliefs, and the noise of social media collide, often leaving shift workers without clear, actionable guidance. Yet, when stripped of the dogma and grounded in the science of circadian biology, nutrition becomes a profoundly powerful and modifiable tool for stabilizing metabolism.

This brings us to exercise, which I argue is the most personal and adaptable lever a shift worker can pull. It doesn't demand perfection, only intention. A single session can alter mood and buffer against depression.[165] Done with consistency, it can improve insulin sensitivity, anchor the circadian system, and extend one's healthspan.[166] For the shift worker, movement isn't just exercise, it's a metabolic intervention and a psychological anchor.

For those battling circadian disruption, the strongest path forward lies in controlling what remains within reach. Since sleep is so often dictated by external forces—the work schedule, the home environment, the inescapable light of day—the real leverage is found in mastering the other two power laws. When used with intention, exercise and nutrition offer a tangible, powerful counterbalance to the physiological strain of a life lived out of sync.

This is not to say that the battle for sleep should be abandoned. But we must be ruthlessly pragmatic. A wellness plan that demands eight perfect hours of sleep from a night-shift nurse with a young family is not a plan; it's a recipe for failure. Here's the core warning: If your plan doesn't fit your real life, it won't bend—it will break you.

When exhaustion mounts and time narrows, rigid expectations around fitness and diet are the first things to collapse, often triggering a spiral of guilt and burnout. The pursuit of perfection becomes counterproductive. A 90-minute gym session may not survive a string of 12-hour shifts, but resistance bands in the breakroom might. Elaborate meal prep may fail, but a commitment to a circadian-aligned eating window is sustainable.

This isn't defeatism, it's biology-aware pragmatism. Health routines must fit the life, not fight it.

You can push through on grit alone. But your body keeps a ledger.

If you remember nothing else from this book, remember this: To survive the physiological toll of shift work, you must respect two biological non-negotiables.

Avoid eating within 3 hours of your intended sleep window.

Late eating disrupts digestion, delays melatonin release, and interferes with the body's natural transition into restorative sleep. Even a small snack can spike insulin and blunt the signal that it's time to rest. Treat your pre-sleep window as a sacred zone for recovery— protect it like your life depends on it, because over time, it might.

Maintain a fasting window of at least 12 hours between your last meal of one shift and the first of the next—16 hours is even more effective.

This fasting window helps realign your metabolic clocks, reduce insulin resistance, and give your body time to reset. It reinforces rhythm in a life that often lacks it. Think of this as a daily metabolic reset button, one that guards against the slow creep of inflammation, weight gain, and fatigue.

Clock Notes

Three Power Laws – A pragmatic health framework for shift workers prioritizing Sleep, Nutrition, and Exercise, ranked by biological impact and practical adaptability.

Movement as Resilience – Exercise serves as both metabolic therapy and emotional buffering; even brief, consistent sessions improve insulin sensitivity and re-anchor biological rhythms.

Biology-Aware Pragmatism – A shift-work health strategy rooted in sustainability; emphasizes fitting routines into real-life constraints rather than enforcing rigid, idealized standards.

Breaking the Seal

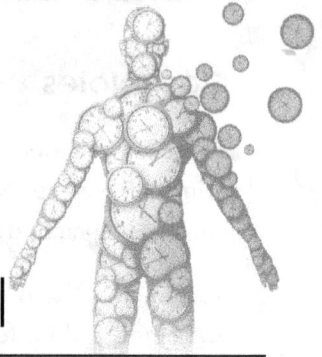

You are human.

Remember that when you're halfway through a 12-hour night shift and feel your physical and mental reserves begin to crumble.

Even the most resilient, disciplined shift worker can be brought to their knees by the biological assault of working against the clock. That's not hyperbole—these shifts can break you.

And this is where we have to talk about discipline. No one is born with an endless supply of it.

Discipline isn't inherited, it's earned. Forged in the quiet moments of preparation. Tested in the crucible of fatigue.

It's a muscle.

And like any muscle, it grows with use, one repetition, one choice, one hard night at a time.

Motivation is a fickle guest.

When motivation leaves, discipline stays.

For the shift worker, the most dangerous part of the night is the final stretch, between 3:00 and 7:00 a.m. This is the circadian nadir, a biological battleground where your cognitive fortitude is at its weakest. Emotional regulation frays. Executive function falters. Blood sugar drops. The vending machine starts to look like an oasis, and your brain, starved for a cheap dopamine hit, begs for the easiest possible win.

This is the moment of truth. I call it breaking the seal.

Once that first impulsive choice is made—the fast-food breakfast on the 7:45 a.m. drive home, the bag of chips you tear into as you walk through the door—the floodgates swing open. This is not a failure of willpower. It's a predictable physiological consequence of circadian misalignment and decision fatigue. Your prefrontal cortex is offline. Your primal brain is in charge.

What prevents this collapse? A system. Not a perfect one, but a practiced one.

A system removes the burden of choice when you're least equipped to make a good one. It's your pre-packed recovery shake. Your no-cook, post-shift meal. Your unwavering "no stopping" rule on the drive home. Your nutritional plan must become a ritual—automatic, rehearsed, and non-negotiable. Like an ACLS algorithm, it shouldn't depend on how you feel. It should kick in because the protocol says so. You don't think. You act.

This is how routine becomes protective. How discipline becomes freedom.

There will be days when the seal breaks. One failure? That's friction. Two? That's risk. Three? That's momentum in reverse. This is the point where momentum either fractures, or fortifies.

Protect the seal, not with perfection, but with consistency. One day off won't hurt you. Two might. Three becomes a pattern.

As you move through this book, remember: evolution didn't design you for this life. But you are not powerless. The protocols within these pages are scaffolds, not salvation. They offer structure and possibility, but the true architect of your health is you. You hold the agency to prepare, to adapt, to begin again.

When your routine cracks, it doesn't mean you've failed. It means you're human.

And humans don't need perfection. They need compassion, consistency, and a system waiting for them when they're ready to step back in.

When you're a shift worker, everything requires intention. Intentionally eating. Intentionally moving. Intentionally resting. In a world turned upside down, intention becomes your compass, restoring rhythm where chaos once reigned.

But intention is only the starting line.

The secret is momentum. And the engine behind it is consistency. Not perfection. Not willpower. Just the repeated choice to show up. Over time, what feels hard becomes habitual. What once demanded effort becomes second nature.

Momentum is your force multiplier—it shapes identity, anchors motion.

But momentum is fragile. In its early stages, it must be protected, like a small flame in the wind. If you build it, guard it. When life interrupts your rhythm—and it will—momentum is what helps you return. It makes beginning again feel less like starting over and more like resuming your path.

In the reality of shift work, momentum is your hidden superpower. Build it with discipline. Sustain it with self-compassion.

There are countless plans out there—protocols, prescriptions, routines—all promising to fix the damage or soften the blow. But before any of them can take hold, before you white-knuckle your way through another "perfect" day, give yourself this: grace.

Though much of this book is rooted in science, real life is not a controlled experiment. There is gray in this work. It's tempting to reduce everything to inputs and outputs. But shift work collides with the unpredictability of human life.

You need a plan. But you also need a plan B.

No single fix will carry you across the finish line. What will is discipline, yes, but also your capacity to endure discomfort, ride out fatigue, and course-correct with compassion when you miss the mark.

You will falter. That is not failure—it is reality. Flexibility is not a flaw in your system. It is the system. Your ability to pivot when control is lost is not weakness—it is wisdom.

There will be nights when you do everything right and still feel broken. Mornings when the best choice is the least perfect one. If shift work fits your life or your financial reality, that is not a moral failing. It is survival.

Extremes are rarely sustainable. Give yourself the space to adapt. The grace to rest without guilt. The courage to begin again without shame.

Discipline will stretch you. Some days, you'll need a nudge. A reset. A reason.

Let this be that reason.

Let this book, this work, be the push that reminds you: you are not alone in this paradox. You are part of a tribe of doers, those who work through the night and undo what the world does not see.

This is not a manifesto. It is an offering, from one shift worker to another.

When you falter, it's not failure—it's part of the rhythm. In shift work, survival isn't a straight line. It's a spiral. You do. You undo. And then, you rise again. That's not weakness. That's adaptation.

We do.

And then we undo.

And then, we rise again.

Clock Notes

Circadian Nadir – The biologically lowest point in alertness, mood, and cognitive performance, typically occurring between 3:00 and 7:00 a.m., where decision fatigue and emotional volatility peak.

Breaking the Seal – A metaphor for the critical moment when a single compromised decision (e.g., poor food choice post-shift) leads to a cascade of behavioral lapses, driven more by biology than willpower.

Momentum Fragility – A recognition that early behavioral momentum is powerful but easily lost; sustaining health gains depends on consistency, not perfection.

When Sleep Fails, Everything Follows

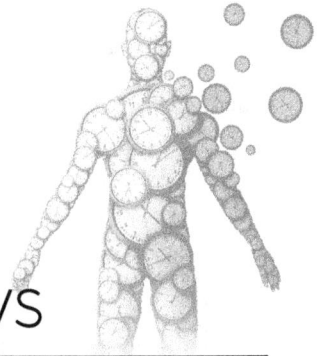

Of the three foundational pillars of health, sleep is the undisputed master. It is a biological necessity, more powerful and restorative than we can possibly measure, a dynamic non-negotiable process that governs cellular repair, hormonal balance, and cognitive function.[167] Yet for the shift worker, this pillar is the first to crumble. A life lived against the clock becomes a life defined by a constant, unwinnable war against sleep.

To understand why this is so damaging, we must first understand the elegant, two-part system that regulates our sleep. Think of it as a biological tug-of-war. On one end of the rope is the homeostatic sleep drive. This is a simple process: the longer you are awake, the more a sleep-promoting chemical called adenosine builds up in your brain, creating a powerful pressure to sleep. This is the "sleep debt" that accumulates with every waking hour.[168]

Pulling on the other end of the rope is the circadian alerting signal. This is the voice of your master clock, the SCN, which sends out a powerful "stay awake" signal throughout the day to counteract the mounting sleep pressure.[169]

In a healthy, synchronized person, these two forces work in perfect harmony. The alerting signal is strongest during the day, keeping you awake and focused. As evening approaches, the alerting signal fades, melatonin begins to rise, and the homeostatic sleep drive finally wins the tug-of-war, pulling you into deep, restorative sleep as the adenosine debt is paid.[170]

For the shift worker, this elegant system collapses. The night shift demands alertness precisely when the circadian "stay awake" signal is at its weakest and the drive to sleep is at its peak. Conversely, the attempt to sleep during the day is a battle against a brain flooded with alerting signals and bathed in environmental light that actively suppresses melatonin. The result is fragmented, low-quality sleep that never fully pays off the homeostatic debt, leading to a state of chronic sleep insufficiency.

And as we've already covered, SWSD, shift work sleep disorder, is the formal diagnosis for a body at war with its own schedule. Its prevalence is staggering.[171]

In one study of nurses, nearly half (44%) of those working shifts met the criteria for probable SWSD.[172] These were often the youngest and least senior nurses, those with fewer external social anchors like marriage or children to help buffer the isolating effects of their work.[173] They suffered from higher rates of insomnia, depression, anxiety, and post-traumatic stress, a psychological toll that mirrored their physiological disruption.[173]

Of course, not everyone is affected in the same way. Your individual chronotype, whether you are a natural "morning lark" or "night owl", plays a significant role. Evening types tend to tolerate night work better, while morning types struggle immensely. Genetic variations, such as in the PER3 gene, also influence our resilience to sleep deprivation.[174] But even for those who seem to adapt, the underlying biological conflict remains.

Sleep loss doesn't just make you tired. Insufficient sleep and circadian misalignment disrupt energy balance, driving an increase in food intake that far outpaces energy expenditure.[175] It impairs cognitive control and heightens the brain's reward sensitivity, making poor food choices nearly inevitable. The neurobehavioral impairment from this chronic sleep debt can be equivalent to alcohol intoxication, making the drive home a life-threatening event.[176]

We tend to think of sleep as a pause, an idle stretch of time where nothing much happens. But the truth is, sleep is the most high-performance maintenance cycle the human body runs. It's not downtime. It's repair time.

When you close your eyes and drift off, your brain doesn't slow down—it shifts gears. Behind the scenes, sleep activates an entire network of genes responsible for healing, hormone regulation, metabolism, and immunity. It's a time when the body performs its most critical restorative work, repairs that don't happen while you're awake.

And in the brain? Something remarkable unfolds.

During sleep, a recently discovered network in the brain called the glymphatic system activates with remarkable precision. It functions less like a car wash and more like an overnight sanitation crew, opening fluid channels between brain cells and mobilizing cerebrospinal fluid to flush out neurotoxic waste, including beta-amyloid and tau proteins implicated in neurodegenerative disease.[177] This cerebral clearance system operates in tandem with slow-wave sleep, when interstitial spaces expand and fluid exchange accelerates.

But here's the critical detail: this process is time-locked to sleep itself. Not just rest, but deep, uninterrupted, circadian-aligned sleep. When sleep is fragmented, shortened, or mistimed, conditions all too common in the life of a night-shift nurse, the glymphatic system can't fully engage. Waste clearance slows. Toxins accumulate. And what starts as mental fog can progress, over years, into measurable cognitive decline.

Researchers now believe this buildup plays a role not just in poor focus or low energy, but in long-term brain health, linking a single night of disrupted sleep to mood disorders, memory loss, and diseases like Alzheimer's.[178]

In rare cases, individuals with a mutation in the ADRB1 gene are able to function on shorter sleep cycles without sacrificing these deep-cleaning processes.[179] Their brains cycle more efficiently. But for most of us, especially those working against the natural rhythm of light and dark, that neuro-cleanup crew gets delayed, disrupted, or dismantled altogether.

And here's the deeper truth: sleep isn't controlled by a single switch or a solitary gene. It's a complex symphony conducted by your internal clocks, shaped by light, food, movement, and rest. Disrupt just one cue, and the entire rhythm can collapse.

Shift work doesn't just interrupt your rhythm, it hijacks it. Sleep is sliced, compressed into unnatural windows, and forced into hours your biology resists. You already know the cost: foggy mornings, restless days, a body that's always running behind.

If you take nothing else from this, remember this: Sleep is the wash cycle for your brain. Miss it, and the grime—the waste, the toxins, the mental fog—doesn't get rinsed away. It lingers. And it builds.

This is the shift worker's paradox in its starkest form. The single most important pillar of health is the one they are forced to sacrifice. While strategies like melatonin supplementation, timed light exposure, and pre-shift naps can help, they are often just scaffolding over a structural fault.[180] This is why mastering the other two power laws, nutrition and exercise, becomes not just a recommendation, but an act of survival.

Clock Notes

Homeostatic Sleep Drive – The pressure to sleep that builds the longer you stay awake, driven by the accumulation of adenosine in the brain.

Glymphatic System – A nighttime waste clearance system in the brain that uses cerebrospinal fluid to flush out toxins like beta-amyloid; optimally activated during deep, circadian-aligned sleep.

ADRB1 Mutation – A rare genetic variant that allows individuals to require less sleep while still achieving adequate neural restoration and glymphatic clearance.

Sleep Debt – The cumulative effect of inadequate sleep that impairs cognitive, emotional, and physiological functioning over time.

Sleep Anchoring – A strategic technique that emphasizes consistent wake times and protective routines to preserve circadian alignment and improve sleep quality, especially in rotating schedules.

Nutrition as a Strategy for Survival

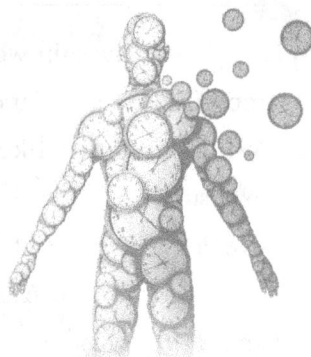

Nutritional strategies for shift workers must prioritize physiology over ideology. This chapter emphasizes foundational choices that support biological resilience, not trends shaped by online narratives.

In a digital age where nutrition has become identity, where phrases like *clean eating, keto warriors, plant-based purity, carnivore diet* and *intuitive eating* carry moral weight, *The Shift Worker's Paradox* offers something different: a pragmatic, biology-based approach designed for those living against their natural circadian rhythm.

Food isn't philosophy—it's fuel, medicine, and metabolic regulation. These online nutrition communities can offer support and inspiration. But they can also promote rigid ideologies that often clash with the biological realities of working nights, rotating shifts, and sleeping during the day.

Among populations vulnerable to metabolic stress—night-shift nurses, emergency responders, and industrial workers—nutrition must prioritize physiology over popularity. Viral trends, no matter how well-intentioned, do not translate universally. Emotionalized food choices, whether rooted in guilt, pride, or tribal loyalty, can worsen fatigue, destabilize glucose levels, and impair cognitive function.

Studies have shown that emotional states and eating styles, such as emotional eating, restrained eating, and external eating, interact with food quality to influence behavior.[181]

Rigid fasting schedules or trend-driven food eliminations can destabilize glucose, especially during overnight hours when energy is critical. Misapplying the concept of "intuitive eating" in the face of disrupted hunger cues may lead to overeating, particularly of ultra-processed, low-nutrient foods.

What follows is a blueprint: pragmatic, adaptable strategies to stabilize metabolism, support alertness, and reduce disease risk. These recommendations are rooted in circadian biology, macronutrient metabolism, and real-world application. What you eat, and when you eat it, can dramatically affect performance and health during shift work.

Meal timing and composition are central. In one study, night-shift workers who consumed a higher-fat, lower-carb meal performed better on cognitive tasks than those who ate a high-carb, low-fat meal.[182] In contrast, carbohydrate-heavy meals consumed close to circadian troughs may impair alertness or spike blood glucose.[183] Night-shift eating often defaults to high-calorie, nutrient-poor foods, disrupting hormones like leptin, ghrelin, and GLP-1, and raising triglycerides and LDL cholesterol.[184]

Snacking, ubiquitous during night shifts, requires special attention. The biological night is a period of impaired glucose tolerance and slower digestion. Large, calorie-dense snacks can worsen fatigue and metabolic strain.[185] Smaller, nutrient-dense options that supply ~10% of daily caloric needs are better tolerated and improve sustained attention.[185] Protein-rich or balanced meals help stabilize glucose and cognitive function throughout the night.[185]

Fat provides energy but may impair alertness when consumed near peak cognitive demands. The timing of fat intake should align with lower-task periods to preserve mental clarity. Workers who bring food from home tend to consume lower-energy-dense options than those relying on canteens or vending machines.[186] Unsurprisingly, vending machine use increases during night shifts.[186]

Snacks should be small, easy to digest, and low in calories. A light snack (~200 kcal) can support alertness without the digestive burden or glucose crash associated with large meals.[187]

The built environment also shapes nutritional behavior. Smart lighting, designated rest areas, and accessible, healthy food options—like fruit baskets or upgraded vending—can reinforce circadian alignment and reduce fatigue.

Social dynamics further influence food choices. Coworker habits, communal stress, and shift culture all shape individual behavior. Interventions like mindfulness training, childcare support, and flexible scheduling have been shown to improve resilience.[188]

Screening for shift tolerance and sleep disorders is essential. Chronotype, personality traits, and family obligations influence adaptability. Tailoring schedules using chronotype data—e.g., avoiding early shifts for evening types—improves sleep and performance.[189] The Munich Chronotype Questionnaire offers a simple tool for aligning schedules with biological preference.[190]

Chrononutrition, the science of how meal timing influences biological rhythms, offers promising strategies. Limiting calorie intake during the circadian night (2:00–5:00 a.m.) while prioritizing meals earlier in the shift supports glucose control.[191] A structured pattern of three meals and two snacks per 24 hours, with lighter meals at night, helps maintain energy without impairing digestion.[191]

Time-restricted eating (TRE) shows metabolic benefits, especially early TRE (calories restricted to the morning and early afternoon).[192] While more research is needed in shift work settings, the principle holds: eating during the biological day is preferable, even if your schedule unfolds at night. Eat early. Eat light. Prioritize protein near the end of your shift.

The composition and timing of calories also matter. Consuming more calories and carbohydrates earlier in the day enhances weight loss and glucose regulation.[193] Even the sequence of macronutrients during meals can affect outcomes; consuming carbohydrates last reduces postprandial glucose in people with prediabetes and type 2 diabetes.[194]

For plant-based shift workers, nutrient quality is key. Protein from tofu, legumes, or quinoa, and healthy fats from nuts or seeds can sustain energy, while fiber-rich whole grains support digestion and glucose regulation. No matter the dietary pattern, the priorities remain the same: nutrient density, appropriate timing, and physiological relevance.

For shift workers, nutrition must be flexible yet foundational. By shifting from emotional allegiance to physiological alignment, nutrition becomes a frontline defense against the strain of working against the clock.

For the shift worker, food is not identity. It is strategy.

While social media debates macronutrient purity, you eat to regulate glucose. To buffer stress. To stay awake when others sleep.

And in that reality, nutrition becomes more than a lifestyle—it becomes a tool. A lever. A countermeasure.

Not every meal will be perfect. Not every shift will go to plan. But each food choice anchored to your biology, not a trend, becomes an act of alignment.

By the time your shift ends and the world winds down, your body is just waking up, hungry, wired, and out of sync. The temptation is real: a heavy meal before collapsing into bed, a midnight snack mid-shift, or a convenience dinner during your commute home. But what if *when* you eat matters just as much as *what* you eat?

Here's the paradox: shift workers don't just eat at odd hours, they eat at biologically *wrong* hours. And this timing doesn't just affect digestion. It alters sleep.

Why? Because your gut and your clock are on different schedules. Digestion slows dramatically at night, and late meals can trigger heartburn, acid reflux, and mid-sleep awakenings that fragment what little rest you're already fighting for.[195] It's not just discomfort—it's disruption.

Emerging research reveals this clearly. One study showed that eating within three hours of bedtime increases the odds of nighttime awakening by nearly 40%, regardless of weight or background.[196] Another found that a high–glycemic index meal eaten four hours before bed actually *improved* sleep onset, while the same meal eaten one hour before bed *delayed* it. Timing matters.[197]

You won't find dozens of randomized trials on meal timing and sleep—they're rare. But the biological cues are there: your metabolism follows a circadian rhythm. And when you force food into a system that's preparing for shutdown, you confuse the clock you're trying to reset.

For the shift worker, this means making peace with a structured rule: cut off meals three hours before sleep, no matter what time that "night" happens to fall. Whether you're turning in at 8 a.m. or 10 p.m., your digestive system needs the same signal your brain does: power down.

This isn't just sleep hygiene. It's circadian nutrition. And in the architecture of shift work recovery, this simple principle may be the lowest-hanging fruit of all.

Eat like you're going to bed soon. Because your biology already is.

Clock Notes

Circadian Night – The biological phase typically aligned with darkness and sleep, during which metabolism slows and digestion becomes less efficient, rendering food intake during this time metabolically disadvantageous.

Macronutrient Sequencing – A nutritional strategy that adjusts the order in which proteins, fats, and carbohydrates are consumed during a meal, with evidence suggesting that consuming carbohydrates last can reduce postprandial glucose spikes.

Biological Fueling – A pragmatic approach to nutrition that prioritizes metabolic function, hormonal balance, and cognitive performance over trends or ideology—especially vital for those working nights or rotating shifts.

Exercise as the
Shift Work Lifeline

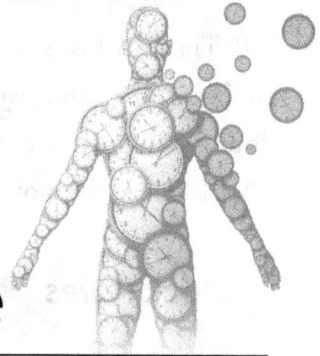

You can't always control your schedule. Or your sleep. But you can move. Restorative sleep is often stolen. But movement remains— portable, flexible, powerful. One of the last reliable tools against the slow erosion of circadian misalignment.

Exercise is physiological intervention.

Hippocrates, often regarded as the father of Western medicine, stated, "Walking is man's best medicine." Thousands of years later, science agrees. Regular movement reduces the risk of diabetes, cardiovascular disease, cancer, obesity, hypertension, depression, and more.[198] And yet, more than 1.8 billion adults fail to meet even minimum activity recommendations.[199] The World Health Organization recommends 150 to 300 minutes of moderate-intensity activity or 75 to 150 minutes of vigorous activity per week.[200] For the shift worker with fragmented time and depleted energy, these goals can feel like fiction.

But unlike sleep, dictated by economic and institutional demands, exercise is adaptable. It may be the most potent of the remaining "power laws." A countermeasure to misaligned rhythms, metabolic dysfunction, and mental fatigue. In this context, movement is not about motivation—it's about reclaiming control.

Shift work imposes chronic biological, psychological, and social strain, increasing the risk of cardiovascular disease, insulin resistance, cognitive decline, and mood disorders.[201] While we have established that sleep disruption lies at the core of these outcomes, physical inactivity, especially in the context of erratic work hours, further amplifies the damage.

Exercise isn't just a routine—it's a strategic intervention. When used wisely, it becomes a tool that spans the full arc of a shift worker's life: before the shift, during the shift, and after the shift

Most shift workers don't hit the gym after a 12-hour night. That's not weakness—it's your biology responding to exhaustion, misaligned rhythms, and depleted reserves. But here's the shift: you don't need hours. Just minutes.

In a study of rotating shift workers, participants performed just 17 minutes of high-intensity training, three times per week. Over eight weeks, they saw measurable improvements in systolic and diastolic blood pressure and HbA1c, key markers for cardiovascular and metabolic health.[202] These improvements occurred even without major changes in body weight or cholesterol.[202] The takeaway is clear: for shift workers, exercise is not about aesthetics. It's about survival.

Short, consistent bouts of movement regulate blood pressure, stabilize glucose, and buffer the toll of sleep disruption.[202] A 10-minute walk. A few bodyweight squats. These micro-interventions stack over time, buffering against the stress of long hours and artificial light.

Timing matters. Exercise just before a night shift has been shown to reduce central systolic blood pressure, arterial stiffness, and vascular risk markers.[203] When paired with post-shift light avoidance, the effects are even more pronounced. This supports the idea that physical activity is not just a cardiovascular tool, but a non-photic zeitgeber, a cue capable of adjusting internal clocks independently of light.[204]

In blind individuals and tightly controlled studies, physical activity alone can entrain melatonin cycles, synchronizing hormonal and metabolic functions even in the absence of daylight.[205]

Beyond its cardiovascular and metabolic impact, physical activity has immediate effects on mental performance. Light to moderate movement, such as walking every 30 minutes during a shift, improves executive function, vigilance, and reaction time.[201] Night-shift workers face compounded cognitive risk: circadian misalignment and accumulated sleep debt. Movement within the shift is one of the few interventions that can immediately blunt these effects.

Back-to-back shifts (or "blocks") bring unique stress. Fatigue builds. Recovery diminishes. Mood and stress tolerance decline. But this is where movement builds more than muscle—it builds resilience.

Exercise between shifts improves sleep quality, mood, and stress resilience.[201] When paired with lighting strategies (e.g., bright light before a night shift, dim environments post-shift), exercise can initiate circadian phase delays that improve overnight performance and next-day recovery.[201] In real-world conditions, where lighting is inconsistent, exercise still helps synchronize peripheral clocks in tissues like liver and muscle.[201]

The third timeline, after the shift, reflects cumulative adaptation. This is where movement becomes a stabilizing habit. Workers who remain physically active across years of shift work report lower rates of depression, burnout, and chronic disease.[206]

Part of this benefit may stem from exercise's effect on the hypothalamic-pituitary-adrenal (HPA) axis. Movement modulates this stress system, dampening overreaction and helping shift workers tolerate long-term biological strain. It also enhances neuroplasticity, supporting emotional flexibility and executive functioning even in the face of chronic circadian disruption.

The perfect plan? It's the one you'll actually follow.

For shift workers, that often means breaking free from rigid models of "working out." It means walking between patient rooms. Taking the stairs. Stretching during change of shift. It means moving when you can, not when it's convenient.

Studies of nurses and industrial workers show that some thrive on structured off-day workouts.[207] Others need flexibility embedded into the shift itself. There's no one-size-fits-all plan. What matters is that it works for you, because what works is what will last.

Sustainable change doesn't begin with intensity. It begins with realism.

Movement isn't just medicine. For the shift worker, it's proof that biology can still be influenced, even when your schedule feels immovable.

Physical activity does more than move muscles—it primes the body for rest. When you exercise, your core temperature rises. But it's the drop that follows, usually 30 to 90 minutes later, that signals your body it's time to sleep.[208] For shift workers navigating misaligned rhythms, this natural cooling effect becomes a powerful cue for rest.

In the end, exercise is your refusal to surrender to the clock. It's your way back to center.

Here's how you can weave it in without leaving the floor:

- 10-Minute Reset Walk → one lap around your unit, warehouse, or worksite at lunch or during charting downtime.

- Hallway Squats → 3 x 30-second bodyweight squats while waiting for labs, a machine cycle, or shift handoff.

- Stair Sprints → 1–2 flights of stairs at moderate pace when moving between departments instead of the elevator.

- Calf Raises → 20 reps while washing hands or waiting for a machine to finish.

- Wall Push-Ups → 10–15 reps in the breakroom or empty hallway—safe, discreet, effective.

- Chair Routine→ sit-to-stand x10 during charting breaks—no gym required.

- Stretch Stack → every 2–3 hours, do:
    - Neck rolls x30 seconds
    - Shoulder shrugs x10
    - Wrist stretches (good for computer/data entry workers)

- Shift Partner Accountability → pair up with a coworker and agree on one *micro-movement cue* (e.g., every time you both leave a patient's room, you do 10 calf raises).

And if you're ready to take it further, if you want maximum return for minimal time, the next chapter introduces the most efficient protocol for metabolic and cognitive resilience.

Clock Notes

Non-Photic Zeitgeber – A time cue (e.g., exercise or meals) that can influence the body's circadian rhythm independent of light exposure, helping regulate internal clocks; critical for shift workers exposed to irregular lighting.

Micro-Interventions – Short, low-barrier bouts of physical activity (e.g., 10-minute walks or squats during shift breaks) that offer measurable cardiovascular, metabolic, and cognitive benefits.

HPA Axis Modulation – The ability of exercise to regulate the hypothalamic-pituitary-adrenal axis, thereby reducing stress reactivity and supporting resilience under chronic biological strain.

Circadian Phase Delay – A shift in the body's biological clock to a later time, which can be achieved through evening exercise and light exposure, used to improve performance during overnight shifts.

Your HIIT Rebellion

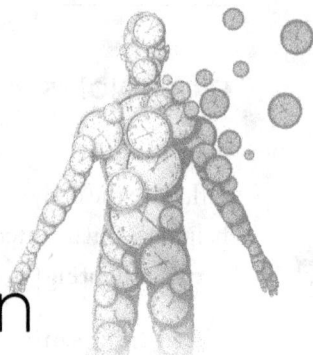

You wake up groggy. The sun's out. But your body still thinks it's 2 a.m. There's laundry to do. Another shift tonight.

Zero time, and even less energy.

The idea of a 60-minute workout? Not just unrealistic.

Laughable.

For shift workers, time isn't just tight. It's fractured. Schedules shift. Recovery slips. Meals answer fatigue, not hunger. Movement fades. And slowly, day by day, the energy you spend outpaces what your body can restore.

The consequences aren't surprising, but they are dangerous: disrupted metabolism, elevated disease risk, and the steady erosion of physical resilience.

Movement matters. It rebuilds what shift work breaks. But at some point, pacing the unit or walking the parking lot after a twelve-hour night isn't enough. Moderate exercise maintains. HIIT rebuilds.

When your rhythms are fractured and your energy runs on fumes, gentle movement only goes so far. The body needs a louder signal, one that cuts through the noise of fatigue and forces your biology to respond.

That's the trap. But there's a tool that works with constraint, not against it: High-Intensity Interval Training (HIIT).

This is your HIIT Rebellion.

HIIT delivers more in less time, perfect for a life that leaves no room for hour-long workouts. In just 15–20 minutes, a wellstructured HIIT session improves insulin sensitivity, lowers BP, and raises BDNF. [209] It's efficient, effective, and essential for cognitive clarity and mood regulation.

HIIT mimics the natural bursts of exertion our bodies evolved for—brief but intense. That burst triggers deeply rooted adaptations: improved glucose control, enhanced stress tolerance, preserved lean mass. [209] Even under conditions of irregular meals, sleep disruption, or long blocks of night shifts, HIIT holds the line.

HIIT simply means pushing above moderate intensity: heart rate, perceived effort, or oxygen use. [209]

Just 2–3 sessions a week, under 20 minutes, can reshape metabolic markers without overhauling your life.

In clinical and occupational settings, HIIT helps address cardiometabolic disease, mitochondrial decline, and the psychosocial effects of chronic stress. [210]

Compared to moderate-intensity continuous training (MICT), HIIT often yields equal or better outcomes in a fraction of the time. [211] HIIT interrupts fatigue. Resets the system.

Studies from Martin Gibala and others demonstrate that four to six 30-second intervals at supramaximal effort, interspersed with 4-minute recovery periods, can match or exceed the benefits of 90 to 120 minutes of continuous moderate exercise. [212]

Even a 10-minute HIIT session can recenter attention, lift mood, and restore a sense of control. [212]

HIIT interventions also enhance autonomous motivation and self-efficacy. Participants report more vitality, less pain, better general health, and improved motivation and stress resilience.[212]

Low-volume HIIT is especially useful for time-strapped workers, but pacing, rest, and appropriate recovery are critical. Too much intensity too often can backfire, reducing adherence and enjoyment.

Avoid HIIT within two hours of planned sleep, especially after night shifts, when recovery is key.[213]

HIIT is a tool, not a mandate.

On days of deep fatigue or emotional depletion, lighter movement—a walk, a stretch, a slow yoga flow—may be the wisest choice.

It gives back something many shift workers feel they've lost: control.

Control over energy. Over biology. Over time.

Because fifteen minutes of effort, in a body pushed to the margins, is not just adaptation.

It's defiance. It's agency. It's a decision to show up when everything else says not to.

Try this: Your HIIT Baseline

- 30 seconds of effort—squats, fast walking, shadowboxing—followed by 90 seconds of rest.

- Repeat 4–6 rounds.

    That's your entry point.
Option 2: The 10-Minute Reset
- 20 seconds of push-ups (modified if needed).

- 40 seconds of rest.

- 20 seconds of air squats.

- 40 seconds of rest.

- 20 seconds of mountain climbers.

- 40 seconds of rest.

- Repeat the cycle 3–4 times.

Option 3: The Shift-Breaker *(perfect for before or after work)*

- 1 minute: jumping jacks (or marching in place).

- 1 minute: rest.

- 1 minute: burpees (or step-backs if lower impact is needed).

- 1 minute: rest.

- 1 minute: alternating lunges.

- 1 minute: rest.

- Repeat 2–3 rounds.

Option 4: The Core Reboot *(low space, high benefit)*

- 30 seconds: plank shoulder taps.

- 30 seconds: rest.

- 30 seconds: glute bridges.

- 30 seconds: rest.

- 30 seconds: bicycle crunches.

- 30 seconds: rest.

- Repeat 3–5 rounds.

These aren't just workouts—they're signals. Each burst tells your biology to adapt, rebuild, and endure. In a world where your schedule fractures time, HIIT makes every minute matter.

Clock Notes

BDNF (Brain-Derived Neurotrophic Factor) – A key neurochemical involved in neuroplasticity, learning, and mood regulation; HIIT has been shown to increase BDNF levels, supporting cognitive clarity and stress recovery.

Supramaximal Intervals – Exercise intervals performed above one's VO_2 max or lactate threshold, often 30 seconds in duration, used in research settings to replicate the benefits of longer-duration moderate exercise in less time.

Metabolic Resilience – The body's capacity to maintain glucose regulation, lean mass, and energy balance under stress; enhanced by HIIT even in the presence of sleep disruption or irregular eating.

The Breakroom: Where Willpower Fades

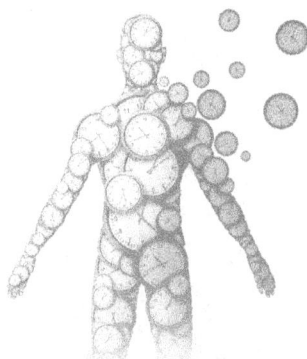

You're sitting alone in the breakroom.

It's 3:12 a.m.

The vending machine hums louder than the clock.

You're not hungry. But something's missing.

You reach for the chips. Not because you need fuel.

Because you need comfort. It's not discipline you're lacking. It's a lifeline.

Shift work does more than disrupt the body's biological rhythms—it fractures the internal compass we rely on to regulate stress, appetite, and emotional equilibrium. While most discussions around shift work focus on its impact on metabolism, cardiovascular risk, and cognitive performance, the emotional terrain remains underexplored. Shift workers face isolation, whether in a hospital breakroom at 3 a.m. or an empty home at 10 a.m., as their schedules push against the rhythms of the broader social structure.

Sleep deprivation impairs the brain's ability to regulate mood and impulse control while heightening the body's inflammatory response.[214] Cortisol rises. Ghrelin increases. Light anchors the

24-hour rhythm. But it's not the only cue. Your rhythms respond to more than sunrise. They shift with reward.

Food. Movement. Sex. Connection. Even substances. Each of these behaviors floods the brain with dopamine, and dopamine, in turn, has the power to reset the clock.[215] These aren't just habits. They're time cues. They shape the rhythms of your brain's reward centers and alter the firing patterns in your suprachiasmatic nucleus, the body's central pacemaker.[215]

When life runs on broken sleep and inverted schedules, these non-light cues can become powerful tools, or hidden disruptors. What you crave isn't just a response to fatigue. It might be your biology, trying to find the rhythm again.

Comfort food becomes therapy because the very neurotransmitters that regulate mood—dopamine, serotonin, norepinephrine—follow rhythms too. And when those rhythms unravel, so does your capacity to cope.[216]

Known in the scientific literature as ego depletion, this concept describes how self-control draws from a limited reservoir of mental energy.

Introduced by psychologist Roy Baumeister, ego depletion suggests that self-discipline wears down with use, much like a muscle.[217]

Shift work doesn't just hijack your schedule—it hijacks your life. It strains relationships. Fractures routines. Steals time. Shift workers tend to be single, participate less in social and cultural activities, and report elevated rates of loneliness.[218] Over time, the cost isn't just logistical—it's emotional.

Mood isn't just circumstance. It's chemistry. And that chemistry runs on rhythm.

Core clock genes—CLOCK, PER2, CRY1, RORA—don't just keep time. They regulate the neurotransmitters that shape how you feel, connect, and cope. When these genes are disrupted, the result isn't just poor sleep. It's mood instability. Irritability. Even symptoms of depression and bipolar disorder. [219]

In the space between duty and depletion, you deserve more than survival.

Systems that support you. Rituals that restore you. Care, without apology.

When the clock pulls you out of rhythm, anchor yourself with one small act.

A breath before the breakroom. A protein bar instead of the chips.

Not for perfection, but for proof that you still get to choose.

Willpower Hacks for Shift Workers

1. Precommit. Decide before fatigue hits. Pack your recovery meal, set your walking shoes out, prep tomorrow's shake. *Systems beat decisions.*

2. If–Then Rules. Write simple triggers: *"If I walk into the breakroom, then I drink water first."* This removes guesswork when your brain is running on fumes.

3. Protect the Seal. Guard the first choice. Say no to the chips at 3 a.m., and it's easier to say yes to breakfast at 8 a.m. Momentum flows forward, or backward.

4. Reduce Friction. Make the good choice the easy one: blackout curtains for sleep, snacks within reach, junk food out of sight. *Exhausted brains choose the path of least resistance.*

5. Fuel Your Brain. Stable glucose = stable decisions. Pair protein with complex carbs instead of chasing sugar spikes that crash your willpower.

6. Anchor with Ritual. Use repeatable cues—music before a workout, one deep breath before bed. Rituals turn discipline into autopilot.

7. Fail Soft, Reset Fast. Slip-ups aren't collapse. Show compassion, reset at the next choice, and move on. *Perfection isn't the goal—consistency is.*

Remember: Willpower isn't infinite. Every choice drains the tank. Build a system so discipline doesn't have to be a fight—it just runs.

Clock Notes

Ego Depletion – A psychological concept describing the reduction of self-control and decision-making capacity after prolonged cognitive or emotional effort; intensified by sleep loss and the chronic strain of shift work.

Dopamine Therapy – The subconscious use of high-reward stimuli (e.g., comfort food, social media, or vending snacks) to stimulate dopamine and soothe emotional fatigue, especially common during circadian lows.

Emotional Dysregulation – Impaired ability to manage mood and stress responses due to circadian misalignment, sleep debt, and neurochemical imbalance, often misinterpreted as weakness or lack of resilience.

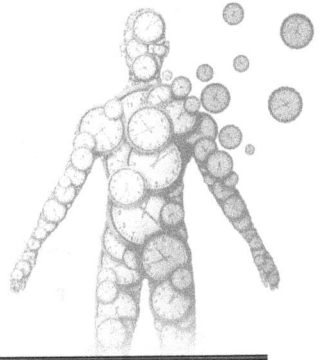

Shielding the Cell

You already know the basics: move, eat well, protect your sleep. But what happens when those aren't enough? When you've done everything right and your body still shows the wear of night shifts and broken rhythms? That's when supplements become more than add-ons, they become quiet allies.

Foundational behaviors—structured movement, circadian-aligned eating, sleep optimization—remain essential. But for many, they're no longer sufficient. This is especially true for those working long rotations, nights without reprieve, or those already showing signs of physiological wear. For these individuals, targeted supplementation may offer an additional layer of protection and recovery.

In the context of shift work, supplements are not quick fixes or performance enhancers. They are tools, meant to buffer the body against predictable strains, support cellular resilience, and bridge unavoidable gaps in rhythm and recovery.

Melatonin, magnesium, adaptogens, and omega-3s, among others, have demonstrated potential in modulating stress pathways, stabilizing mood, promoting sleep depth, and reducing inflammation.[220] Vitamins D and B, complex vitamins supporting energy metabolism and immune function, two pillars that often weaken under artificial light exposure, irregular eating, and fragmented rest.[221]

This section explores evidence-based supplementation strategies designed to support the three foundational Power Laws of Health: Sleep, Nutrition, and Exercise.

Each chapter moving forward draws on current research and integrates real-world considerations—like dosing, timing, tolerability, accessibility, and cost.

The goal isn't to overwhelm with options. It's to empower with understanding. To help shift workers make informed, strategic choices based on their unique schedules, symptoms, and biology.

These compounds are safe, well-tolerated, and backed by evidence for everyday use. They're not performance-enhancers or emergency fixes—they're quiet allies, working in the background to recalibrate your biology.

Their purpose is rhythm. Depth. Repair.

Think of them as biological scaffolding, tools that stabilize your system so that when everything else gets pulled off-center, your body can still find its way back.

Let's be honest: supplements can get expensive. And while foundational support is powerful, not every shift worker has the luxury of filling a cabinet with capsules and powders.

That's why this section doesn't list everything that might help.

It highlights what matters most, especially when decisions matter more than abundance.

It highlights what matters most, especially if you need to make choices.

Clock Notes

Mitochondrial Efficiency – The ability of mitochondria to produce energy (ATP) effectively; compromised by circadian misalignment, leading to fatigue, metabolic dysfunction, and impaired cellular repair.

Oxidative Stress – An imbalance between free radicals and antioxidants in the body, worsened by poor sleep, inflammation, and night shift exposure, contributing to aging and chronic disease.

Adaptogens – Plant-based compounds (e.g., ashwagandha, rhodiola) that help modulate the stress response and stabilize mood, energy, and immune function in biologically demanding conditions.

PART I

Foundational Support – Stability in an Unstable System

A Compass in the Dark

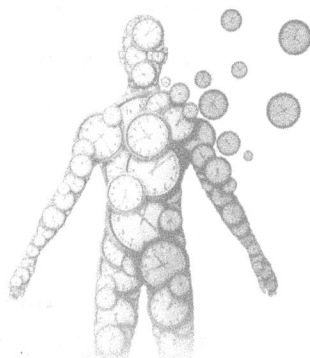

It's 8:12 a.m. The blinds are drawn, but light leaks through. You've been off shift for over an hour, but your body won't shut down.

You scroll your phone, too wired to sleep, too tired to be awake.

This is where melatonin begins. Or where it should have.

Melatonin, often called the "hormone of darkness," plays a critical role in synchronizing the body's internal clock with the environmental light-dark cycle.[222] Produced by the pineal gland in response to darkness, melatonin signals the onset of biological night and initiates time-of-day-specific processes throughout the body.[222]

When circulating melatonin levels surpass a certain threshold, the brain and body interpret this as night. When levels fall below this threshold, the biological day resumes.

Up to one-third of night-shift workers report nonrestorative sleep.[223] Unlike typical insomnia, they attempt rest when melatonin levels are low and alerting signals rise, in broad daylight, when the body promotes wakefulness.

Melatonin extends far beyond sleep, regulating cardiovascular, reproductive, and metabolic systems while acting as a powerful antioxidant and neuroendocrine modulator.[224]

In one randomized controlled trial, melatonin users showed an 80% increase in DNA repair activity during daytime sleep compared to placebo, a direct counter to the oxidative damage shift work accelerates. [225]

This matters. Shift work is a probable carcinogen, in part because melatonin, the hormone that signals night, is suppressed. An ancient survival signal silenced by fluorescent light.

Reduced melatonin secretion, whether from artificial light or circadian misalignment, is associated with insulin resistance and type 2 diabetes. [226] For morning types on night shifts, or anyone under bright light, melatonin output drops even further. [227]

Melatonin isn't a sedative. When timed correctly, it can shift the circadian clock, advancing or delaying biological time to help shift workers adapt. [224]

Take a nurse preparing for three consecutive night shifts. To shift their internal rhythm and improve nighttime alertness, they take 0.5 to 3 mg of melatonin between 6:00 and 8:00 a.m. on the day before their first night shift. This early biological morning dose helps delay the circadian clock. Later that day, they nap from 2:00 to 4:00 p.m. before reporting for a 7:00 p.m. shift.

After each night shift ends around 7:30 a.m., they take melatonin 30 minutes before their intended daytime sleep. The room is dark. Quiet. Cool. Melatonin signals rest, even in daylight.

This isn't hypothetical—controlled studies confirm the effect.

Studies using low-dose, fast-release melatonin (1–3 mg) show improved sleep latency, total sleep time, and subjective sleep quality during daytime rest. [228]

Despite robust evidence, melatonin remains underused among shift workers. Product quality varies. Slow-release formulas often linger too long, while fast-release versions more closely mimic the body's natural melatonin spike. Over-the-counter access doesn't ensure effective use: dose, timing, and formulation all matter.

To be effective, melatonin must be timed precisely, ideally taken after a night shift but far from any safety-sensitive operational window. Combined with light therapy, post-shift darkness, and timed caffeine, melatonin becomes part of a larger circadian strategy.

Melatonin won't undo circadian chaos, but it helps repair what misalignment leaves behind. The gap between research and practice remains, and shift workers continue to navigate complexity with vague advice and inconsistent products. That must change.

As evidence grows, melatonin should no longer be treated as an optional aid. For shift workers, it is a biological tool for sleep, repair, and disease prevention.

Melatonin doesn't just signal rest—it signals recovery. It restores rhythm, reduces strain, and rewrites the story of fatigue.

Blueprint Supplement Protocol: Melatonin

Category: Function Support (Circadian Realignment)

Form: Fast-release melatonin (0.3–3 mg) is optimal for circadian signaling. Avoid extended-release unless managing diagnosed sleep phase disorders.

Timing:

- To support post-shift daytime sleep: take 30–60 minutes before sleep, typically around 8:00–9:00 a.m.

- To shift your biological clock ahead of a night shift block: take 0.5–3 mg between 6:00–8:00 a.m. the day before your first night shift to delay circadian onset.

Onset: Effects begin within 30–60 minutes; peak levels reached within 1–2 hours depending on absorption and formulation.

Duration: Best used in 3–5 day blocks during shift transitions. Continuous long-term use may reduce sensitivity and should be cycled or reassessed.

Pairing:

- Optimize with blackout curtains, blue light blocking glasses, and cool, quiet sleep settings.

- Pair with pre-shift light exposure and morning darkness post-shift to amplify circadian adaptation.

Small Compounds, Big Shifts

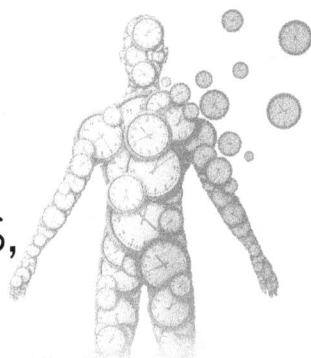

It's 6:30 a.m. You've just finished a 12-hour shift, and now you're staring at the ceiling in a dark room, waiting for sleep that won't come. You've tried melatonin. Blackout curtains.

White noise.

And still, your brain won't quiet down.

This is where amino acids may help, not as knockout drugs, but as quiet allies in circadian repair. Among the foundational elements of nutrition, amino acids shape muscle repair, support metabolic health, and drive neurotransmitter synthesis.[229]

But for shift workers navigating disrupted circadian rhythms, certain amino acids may offer more than structural or metabolic value—they may influence the sleep-wake cycle itself.

They don't sedate. They recalibrate. Not by force, but by working *with* your biology, helping it find its way back.

This emerging intersection of amino acid metabolism and circadian biology opens new, practical avenues for targeted supplementation.

Take L-tryptophan, a well-established precursor to melatonin. Research shows a temporal relationship between tryptophan levels and melatonin production.[230]

In infant studies, nighttime formula enriched with L-tryptophan supported more consolidated sleep-wake patterns.[231]

In shift workers, nighttime supplementation may enhance melatonin synthesis and promote better daytime sleep.

In adults, daily doses of around two grams have shown mild improvements in sleep parameters.[232]

While not a hypnotic, L-tryptophan supports the body's own sleep systems. Still, no strong evidence confirms it shifts the circadian phase.

More promising is L-serine. In animals, it amplified the circadian phase-shifting effect of light by 86%.[233]

In humans, taken before bed, it may enhance light's ability to advance the clock.

That matters for shift workers trying to reset after rotating shifts or long night runs.

L-ornithine takes a different path. Not a phase-shifter, but a resilience booster.

Early studies suggest that 400 mg daily may improve sleep quality under stress and even delay melatonin rhythm onset.[234]

A 15-minute melatonin delay might seem small, but for shift workers, small changes matter.

The studies had limitations—light, food timing, and sleep environment were not controlled.

Still, these findings open new doors.

Then there's L-glycine. Safe. Cheap. Widely available.

Taken one hour before bed, 3 grams can shorten sleep latency, improve efficiency, and reduce next-day fatigue, even under partial

SMALL COMPOUNDS, BIG SHIFTS

sleep restriction.[235] Its mechanism involves the suprachiasmatic nucleus, the body's central clock.

For those recovering on broken sleep or fighting through circadian misalignment, glycine may help stabilize sleep architecture.[235]

They don't override. They attune. They don't knock you out—they ease you in.

They are gentle nudges, not hammers.

Subtle support. Biological alignment. Low risk, high relevance.

The evidence is early. Most studies lack controls for light exposure, temperature, or meal timing. Few examine combinations with melatonin or light therapy.

But these gaps suggest future opportunity, not futility.

For now, shift workers looking for low-cost strategies might consider L-tryptophan, L-serine, L-ornithine, or L-glycine.

Timed correctly—and combined with strategic sleep hygiene, meal timing, and light control—they may deliver real-world gains.

They don't solve the paradox of shift work, but they offer leverage. Small, precise levers that, when timed right, can shift biology back toward balance.

Amino Acids: The Evidence Ladder

Tier 1 – Strongest Evidence

- **L-Glycine**

    o Dose: ~3 g, 1 hour before sleep

    o Effects: Shortens sleep latency, improves efficiency, reduces next-day fatigue, even under restricted sleep.

    o Mechanism: Acts on the suprachiasmatic nucleus, stabilizing the body's master clock.

    o Verdict: Safe, cheap, widely available—best current option for shift workers.

Tier 2 – Moderate Evidence
- **L-Tryptophan**
  - Dose: ~2 g daily
  - Effects: Precursor to melatonin; supports natural sleep processes and may improve daytime sleep after night shifts.
  - Limitations: Mild effects; no strong evidence it shifts circadian phase.
  - Verdict: Gentle support for melatonin pathways; worth trying, but results are subtle.

Tier 3 – Early/Experimental Evidence
- **L-Serine**
  - Dose: Experimental (studies limited)
  - Effects: In animals, enhances the phase-shifting effect of light by ~86%. In humans, may help reset the body clock when combined with timed light.
  - Verdict: Promising but unproven, works best as part of a *light-plus-supplement* strategy.

- **L-Ornithine**
  - Dose: ~400 mg daily
  - Effects: Improves perceived sleep quality under stress; may delay melatonin onset by ~15 minutes.
  - Limitations: Small effect size; studies lacked environmental controls.
  - Verdict: A "resilience booster," not a true clock-shifter.

Blueprint Supplement Protocol: Amino Acids for Circadian Recovery

Category: Foundational Support (Sleep, Stress, and Circadian Repair)

Form: Use pure amino acid powders or capsules, either as individual agents or stacked formulations. Focus on glycine, L-tryptophan, L-serine, and L-ornithine for circadian recovery and restorative sleep.

Timing:

- L-glycine: 3 g taken 1 hour before intended sleep, especially after night shifts or on off-days.

- L-tryptophan: 1–2 g taken 30–60 minutes before bedtime to support melatonin synthesis.

- L-serine: 3 g before bed, particularly on days with planned morning light exposure (to enhance phase advance).

- L-ornithine: 400 mg in the evening after the final shift of a block, to support cortisol downregulation and sleep depth.

Onset:

- Glycine and tryptophan often show benefits within 1–2 nights.

- L-serine may require up to one week, especially when paired with light therapy.

- L-ornithine may improve emotional recovery and next-day energy within several days.

Pairing:

- Combine L-serine with bright morning light for circadian phase shifting.

- Use L-glycine and L-tryptophan together on post-shift or recovery days for synergistic sleep support.

- Pair L-ornithine with magnesium glycinate for enhanced stress-buffering and parasympathetic recovery.

The Sun You Can Swallow

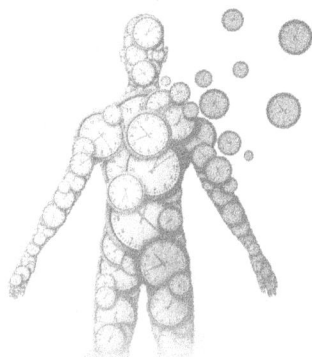

It's 4:00 p.m., and you've just woken up after a night shift. You haven't seen sunlight in two days. Your bones ache. Your sleep feels shallow. Your mood? A little off.

What's missing isn't just rest—it's light. And the molecule that light was supposed to give you: vitamin D3.

In a world where night replaces day and fluorescent corridors stand in for sunlight, shift work quietly dismantles your body's access to its primary source of vitamin D.

And here's the truth: It's not just a vitamin. It's a hormone. A synchronizer. A signal from the sun.

Synthesized in the skin, it triggers cascades that influence immunity, metabolism, and mood.[236]

Yet for those working in darkness or sleeping through daylight, deficiency becomes a silent, cumulative risk. Vitamin D3 influences circadian function through its receptors in brain regions that regulate the sleep–wake cycle.[236] For shift workers, this isn't a marginal concern—it's built into the job.

A comprehensive meta-analysis confirms what clinical intuition has long suspected: shift workers exhibit lower serum 25-OH-D levels compared to non-shift workers.[237]

The mechanism is clear—decreased sunlight exposure, disrupted eating patterns, and lower intake of fortified foods contribute to insufficient vitamin D synthesis and absorption. [237]

The consequences extend beyond skeletal health.

Low vitamin D levels are associated with increased risk of autoimmune disease, cardiovascular events, neuropsychiatric disorders, metabolic dysfunction, and impaired sleep regulation.[238]

Dietary sources like egg yolks, fatty fish, and organ meats offer small amounts, but they're not enough.

It begins in the skin, where UVB transforms cholesterol into the raw material. The liver shapes it. The kidneys finish it. Together, they create the active hormone that regulates calcium, immunity, and rhythm.

In shift workers, limited exposure to natural light disrupts this entire regulatory cascade.

Poor dietary intake.

Inconsistent supplement adherence.

And body fat that hoards the nutrient like a miser traps gold.

The result: low circulating levels, disrupted calcium homeostasis, increased inflammation, and worsening of sleep and mood symptoms already aggravated by shift work. [235]

Low vitamin D is linked to poor sleep quality, longer sleep latency, and even shift work sleep disorder.[235]

By impacting serotonin and melatonin pathways, deficiency erodes circadian stability.

Beyond sleep, vitamin D status influences cardiovascular and skeletal resilience.

Meta-analyses link low D levels to higher cardiovascular mortality and worse lipid profiles.[239] For female shift workers, elevated bone turnover suggests a connection to increased fracture risk. Routine screening and correction should be part of occupational health protocols, especially for shift workers.

But challenges persist.

Studies vary. Definitions differ. Supplementation habits fluctuate across seasons and sexes. Still, consensus targets remain: maintain 25-OH-D levels above 20 ng/mL, with adjustments based on individual factors.[240]

Supplementation is simple, cost-effective, and scalable.

Take D3 with dietary fat to enhance absorption. Most adults benefit from 1,000–2,000 IU daily.

Higher if deficiency is confirmed. In a life shaped by artificial light and circadian disarray, vitamin D3 becomes more than a bone-health supplement.

It becomes a proxy for light.

A hormone of harmony.

A molecule of time itself.

Correcting D3 isn't just preventative medicine.

It's an act of reconnection—with light, with rhythm, with the body's forgotten language of day and night.

Vitamin D3 & Shift Work: Evidence Hierarchy

Strong Evidence

Bone Health: Vitamin D3 deficiency leads to impaired calcium homeostasis, bone loss, and increased fracture risk, especially in female shift workers with elevated bone turnover.[241]

Cardiovascular Mortality: Meta-analyses consistently link low vitamin D levels with higher risk of cardiovascular events and death.[242]

Moderate Evidence

Sleep Quality & Circadian Stability: Deficiency is associated with poor sleep efficiency, longer sleep latency, and worse outcomes in shift work sleep disorder. Mechanisms likely involve serotonin and melatonin pathways.[243]

Mood & Neuropsychiatric Disorders: Observational data link low vitamin D with depression and cognitive decline, but causality remains debated.[244]

Emerging Evidence

Autoimmune Disorders: Low vitamin D status correlates with increased autoimmune disease risk (e.g., multiple sclerosis, type 1 diabetes), though shift-work–specific data are limited.[245]

Metabolic Dysfunction: Associations with obesity and insulin resistance are biologically plausible, but results across studies remain inconsistent.[246]

Blueprint Supplement Protocol:
Vitamin D3 (Cholecalciferol)

Category: Foundational Support (Immune, Mood, and Circadian Health)

Form: Fat-soluble secosteroid hormone, typically found in softgels, capsules, or liquid drops.

- Vitamin D3 (cholecalciferol) is preferred over D2 for superior potency and bioavailability.

Dosing:

- General maintenance: 1,000–2,000 IU daily for most adults.

- Deficiency correction: 5,000 IU daily for 8–12 weeks under clinical supervision.

- Periodic lab monitoring (25(OH)D) is advised, especially for shift workers at risk for deficiency due to limited sun exposure.

Timing:

- Take with your largest fat-containing meal of the day, morning or evening, based on your shift pattern.

- Consistency matters more than clock time.

Onset:

- Serum vitamin D levels typically improve over 4–12 weeks.

- Clinical effects (mood elevation, immune resilience, sleep regulation) may emerge gradually during this window.

Pairing:

- Combine with magnesium (essential for vitamin D metabolism),

- Vitamin K2 (to support calcium routing to bones and away from arteries), and

- Omega-3 fatty acids (for anti-inflammatory and circadian rhythm synergy).

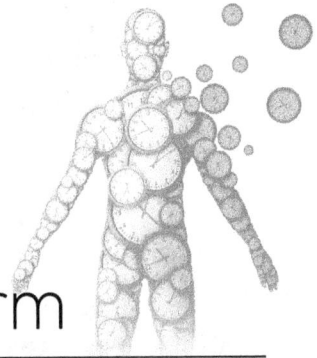

Stability in the Storm

The night is over, but your brain isn't. You're off shift, but wired. The cortisol spike hasn't faded. Your thoughts race. Sleep feels far away.

Your body's rhythm is misfiring. And it's not just about melatonin—it's about recovery. This is where omega-3s may help, not to induce sleep, but to calm the system behind it.

Among the nutritional strategies available to support shift workers, omega-3 fatty acids stand out for their multi-system benefits.

Omega-3 fatty acids, especially EPA and DHA, offer compelling benefits for shift workers navigating cognitive fatigue, emotional burnout, and the physiological strain of circadian disruption.[247]

They don't sedate. They stabilize.

Omega-3s contribute to shift work adaptation by modulating stress responses, stabilizing mood, and regulating cortisol dynamics, benefits that extend beyond their well-known cardiovascular and anti-inflammatory effects. In a randomized controlled trial among nurses, supplementation with omega-3 polyunsaturated fatty acids (O3PUFAs) led to significant reductions in morning cortisol levels and subjective symptoms of burnout.[248]

The relationship between cortisol and burnout wasn't linear, suggesting omega-3s may work not by suppressing stress outright, but by restoring rhythm and hormonal sensitivity.[248]

The body cannot produce omega-3s on its own. You must consume them, through diet or supplements. Fatty fish like salmon and sardines remain the gold standard, but high-quality fish oil or algal oil supplements offer practical options.

For shift workers, EPA may blunt the inflammatory consequences of chronic stress.

DHA supports clarity, cognitive recovery, and mental sharpness under strain.

But here's what the labels miss, and what shift workers need to know.

To achieve an omega-3 index of around 8%—a level associated with a five-year increase in life expectancy—supplementation with at least 2 grams per day is often required.[249] Most Americans hover around 4–5%, especially if they don't consume fish regularly.[249] The form matters too: triglyceride-based supplements are more bioavailable than ethyl ester forms and should always be taken with food for optimal absorption.[250]

Omega-3s don't just buffer stress—they may protect the brain from what happens when recovery is skipped too often. DHA, in particular, shows promise in improving sleep quality and limiting the damage of fragmented or insufficient rest.[249]

Neurodegenerative diseases like Alzheimer's don't start with memory loss. They begin quietly, years earlier, with the breakdown of brain maintenance systems.

Dementia progression has been linked to glymphatic dysfunction and microvascular changes, both of which may be positively influenced by omega-3 PUFAs.[251] These essential fats are more than structural components of the brain; they exhibit anti-inflammatory effects, support microvascular health, and may enhance glymphatic clearance. In this way, omega-3s don't just offer protection. They offer housekeeping.

In the chaos of shift work, where light, sleep, and meals fall out of sync, this matters more than we realize. Because neuroprotection isn't just about aging. It's about function. Focus. Emotional regulation. Repair.

In a system that pushes you to your edge, and then asks for more, omega-3s aren't a luxury.

They can't undo the night shift. But they can steady you within it, protecting your brain, your focus, and your future.

Blueprint Supplement Protocol:
Omega-3 Fatty Acids (EPA + DHA)

Category: Foundational Support (Inflammation, Mood, and Neurovascular Health)

Form: Use high-purity triglyceride-form fish oil or algal oil (for plant-based users), ensuring a strong EPA + DHA profile.

- Triglyceride forms have superior absorption compared to ethyl esters.

- Verify third-party testing for purity, oxidation levels (TOTOX), and heavy metals.

Dosing:

- Aim for 2,000–3,000 mg of combined EPA/DHA daily to reach an omega-3 index ≥8%, a level linked to longer lifespan, reduced inflammation, and improved heart-brain function.

- Individuals with high inflammatory load or mood concerns may benefit from doses on the higher end of this range.

Timing:

- Take with a fat-containing meal for improved bioavailability, especially critical for ethyl ester forms.

- Split dosing (e.g., morning and evening) supports stable plasma levels and enhances GI tolerance.

Onset:

- Anti-inflammatory and mood benefits may begin within 2–4 weeks.

- Neurovascular and cellular membrane integration builds over several months, supporting long-term resilience.

Pairing:

- Combine with saffron to amplify neurovascular effects and mood regulation.

- Stack with phosphatidylserine to support cortisol rhythm, executive function, and cognitive recovery during shift transition.

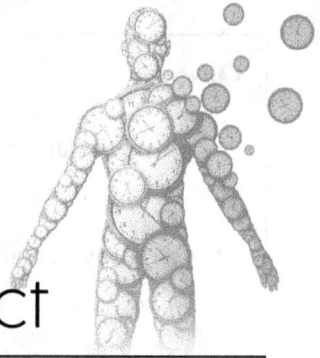

The Silent Architect

Your body feels tired, but your mind won't power down. You're wired. Restless. Mentally buzzing when all you want is sleep. Magnesium won't knock you out. But it will slow the system. It quiets the noise. Calms the current.

And helps bring the body back into rhythm—gently, quietly, consistently.

Magnesium is one of the body's most essential yet underappreciated elements, crucial for more than three hundred enzymatic reactions, yet under-consumed by a substantial portion of the adult population.[252]

For shift workers, disrupted sleep, elevated stress, and altered hormonal rhythms challenge physiological balance.

Magnesium supports this balance by stabilizing biochemical pathways and buffering neurophysiological strain.

It doesn't override. It restores.

Systematic reviews have revealed a growing body of evidence linking magnesium to improved sleep patterns, reduced anxiety, and better regulation of stress-related biomarkers.[253]

While observational studies report associations between magnesium status and sleep quality—including reductions in nighttime awakenings, improved sleep latency, and reduced daytime sleepiness—clinical trials offer mixed results. [253]

Yet one theme persists: higher doses and more absorbable forms work best, especially for those with poor baseline sleep or elevated anxiety.[254]

Magnesium regulates circadian and neurochemical processes through direct physiological pathways.[253]

As a natural NMDA receptor antagonist, magnesium tempers neural excitability, reducing nighttime restlessness and promoting slow-wave (deep) sleep.[255]

Its partial agonist action at GABA-A receptors promotes calm without causing sedation and supports sleep without suppressing natural rhythms.[255]

Rodent studies show that magnesium depletion results in fragmented sleep and increased stress responsiveness, while supplementation restores circadian rhythm integrity and behavioral stability.[256]

In humans, these mechanisms translate into clinical effects: trials report improved sleep quality with forms such as magnesium oxide, citrate, and aspartate when dosed at or above 300 mg of elemental magnesium.[257]

In 2010, a novel compound, magnesium L-threonate (Magtein®), was developed and shown to elevate magnesium levels in the brain and neurons.[257]

Support, not sedation.

Magnesium's role in stress physiology is compelling.

It modulates the HPA axis and may help restore normal cortisol rhythms, a central concern in shift workers with burnout. [256]

Magnesium paired with vitamin B6 reduces anxiety symptoms more than magnesium alone.[258] B6 supports neurotransmitter synthesis, enhancing magnesium's effects.

The combination appears effective in reducing generalized anxiety and tension-related symptoms.

Form matters as much as timing.

Inorganic magnesium oxide, though used, is less bioavailable than organic salts such as magnesium glycinate or threonate.[259]

Magnesium's effects are also dose-dependent—studies using less than 100 mg of elemental magnesium per day report minimal benefits, while those using 300 mg–700 mg tend to show improvements in both mood and sleep parameters. [253]

Evening or bedtime dosing appears more effective for sleep support, aligning with natural circadian rhythms.

Precision matters. But in magnesium's case, absorption matters more.

Social media and public interest have fueled a resurgence of attention to magnesium as a natural sleep aid, but with that popularity comes misinformation.

Anecdotal claims often outpace the clinical data, and patients present having self-supplemented without understanding dose, form, or potential interactions.

Nevertheless, magnesium remains one of the safest, most tolerable over-the-counter options available for addressing the physiological wear of shift work.

For the shift worker lying awake despite exhaustion, for the parent doing bedtime after a night shift, for the clinician holding chaos inside while appearing composed, magnesium offers a quiet kind of rescue.

It doesn't make the world less demanding. But it helps your system absorb the demand without breaking. For shift workers, magnesium is less about sedation, and more about synchronization. A stabilizer for a world that won't slow down.

Blueprint Supplement Protocol: Magnesium

Category: Foundational Support (Sleep Depth, Stress Modulation, and Cellular Stability)

Form: Choose magnesium glycinate for relaxation and sleep, magnesium L-threonate (Magtein®) for cognitive and neural support, or magnesium citrate for general replenishment and digestive motility.

- Avoid magnesium oxide, which has low bioavailability and limited therapeutic effect.

Dosing:

- 300–700 mg/day of elemental magnesium, adjusted based on individual needs, stress burden, and symptom severity.

- Monitor for GI tolerance; divide doses if necessary to avoid loose stools.

Timing:

- Evening or pre-sleep dosing enhances sleep latency, depth, and circadian alignment.

- Split dosing (morning and night) may support stress buffering across the shift cycle.

Onset:

- Subjective improvements in sleep and relaxation often appear within 7–10 days.

- Deeper circadian and mood-regulating effects build over 3–6 weeks of consistent use.

Pairing:

- Combine with vitamin B6 (25–50 mg) to enhance neurotransmitter synthesis (e.g., GABA, serotonin).

- Stack with L-theanine, glycine, or apigenin for synergistic parasympathetic activation and nervous system down-shifting.

Resetting The Clock: Tools That Don't Come in a Bottle

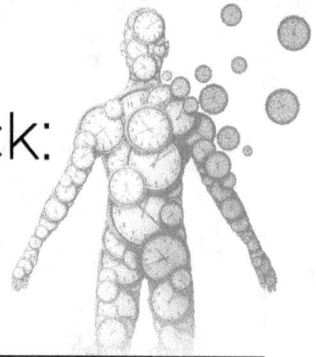

At 3:40 a.m., the ICU is quiet, but never still.

Under the flicker of fluorescents, a nurse pulls back from the desk, eyelids dragging, reaching for a second cup of coffee—enough to stay upright, but not aligned.

This is the life of the night shift: awake, alert, but often out of rhythm. And in this world, the most effective interventions don't sedate or stimulate—they restore balance.

While medications are sometimes necessary, nonpharmacologic strategies remain the first line of defense in managing shift work sleep disorder. They address the underlying misalignment between the body's internal clock and the external demands of a shifted life, offering a path back to synchrony without the side effects of pharmacologic sedation or stimulation.

Central among these strategies are naps and timed light exposure, both supported by decades of research and endorsed by clinical guidelines from the American Academy of Sleep Medicine (AASM).[260] When implemented, these interventions improve alertness, reaction time, and overall performance—key metrics for shift workers whose errors can carry disproportionate consequences.

Among these tools, two stand out not just for their impact, but for how often they're misunderstood.

Napping, often dismissed as fatigue mismanagement, is in fact a physiological tool for alertness optimization. Short naps taken before or during a shift—around 20 minutes—can improve vigilance, reduce errors, and blunt the decline in cognitive function that accumulates across nocturnal hours.[261] Unlike full sleep episodes, strategic naps restore alertness and motor coordination without triggering deep sleep inertia. They offer a targeted reset, a physiological reboot designed for utility, not depth.

Bright light, when timed, triggers both a rise in alertness and a shift in the body's internal clock. Exposure above 5,000 lux suppresses melatonin, raises core body temperature, and sharpens mental focus.[262] When administered during the night shift, light exposure can push the circadian clock forward, helping to delay the sleep phase and improve alignment with nocturnal work.[262] Light becomes a drug, and timing becomes the dosage. Misuse, such as exposure to bright screens too close to sleep, can further disrupt rhythms, while precision enhances adaptability.

Together, naps and light form a simple but powerful toolkit, resetting physiology without medication.

When combined, these interventions may be more powerful than either alone. In a pilot study involving professional drivers working back-to-back 24-hour shifts, a dual protocol of two 20-minute naps followed by 10-minute exposures to bright light reduced objective measures of sleepiness behind the wheel.[263] Although subjective sleepiness scores remained unchanged, physiological data captured via polysomnography showed meaningful reductions in drowsiness.[263] This discrepancy underscores an important reality in shift work: how you feel is not always how your brain performs. Objective readiness can rise even when the body still signals fatigue.

None of this is meant to suggest that naps and light therapy are always realistic. Many shift workers, especially in healthcare, don't have the luxury of controlled environments, scheduled breaks, or consistent lighting conditions. Some work in windowless units. Others go entire nights without a moment to pause. And for parents, caregivers, or those balancing multiple jobs, "timing light" can feel laughable.

But here's the truth: the utility of these tools doesn't always lie in their perfect execution. Sometimes, their value is in the understanding they offer.

Understanding that alertness is not just about willpower—it's about physiology. That the dip you feel at 4:00 a.m. isn't weakness— it's a drop in core body temperature and a surge in melatonin. That the post-shift crash isn't failure—it's a mismatch between your biology and your obligations.

When you understand the mechanisms—what the body is trying to do, and why—it becomes easier to meet yourself with grace instead of judgment. And it becomes easier to make small, strategic shifts where possible: a 10-minute light exposure instead of none. A 15-minute rest instead of scrolling. Dimming lights after work instead of blasting blue light.

Even imperfect strategies can carry power, not because they fix everything, but because they represent a reclaiming of rhythm, one choice at a time.

These strategies demand more than knowledge—they require structure. Protect brief naps when possible. Time light exposure to be short and intense, enough to reset the clock without sabotaging post-shift sleep. Apply both proactively, before fatigue takes hold, not just in response to it. When combined with good sleep hygiene, dietary awareness, and scheduled recovery periods, these interventions create the foundation of circadian resilience, a blueprint for sustaining health in a schedule that was never meant to be sustainable.

In a world built on pharmaceutical shortcuts, nonpharmacologic strategies face a harder truth: You can't outsource sleep—you have to restore it yourself. And for the shift worker, that restoration doesn't begin in a bottle. It begins in rhythm—reclaimed one choice, one light, one pause at a time.

PART II

Targeted Support – Precision in the Midst of Chaos

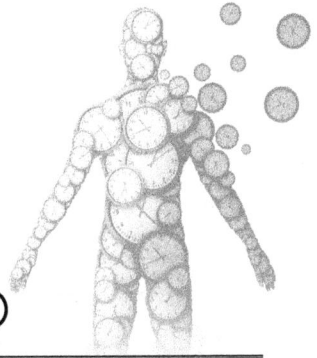

The Caffeine Trap

It's 3:45 a.m.

The emergency department is chaos, but your brain is louder.

You sip your second energy drink, the one you swore you wouldn't need. You're not chasing clarity.

You're chasing consciousness. Again.

Caffeine is the most consumed psychoactive substance in the world, used by over 85% of U.S. adults and often regarded as an essential coping mechanism for fatigue among shift workers.[264] It sharpens focus. Elevates mood. Improves reaction time.[265]

In the context of sleep deprivation and circadian misalignment, its stimulant properties become a default remedy. But for shift workers, caffeine is more than a lifeline—it's a liability when mistimed.

By antagonizing adenosine receptors, caffeine delays sleep pressure and promotes wakefulness.[266] Doses between 200 mg and 600 mg improve performance in monotonous tasks, especially under sleep-deprived conditions. It enhances strength, endurance, and reaction time.[266]

But the benefits are highly time-dependent. Caffeine taken around midnight may extend function into the early hours of a shift. But with a half-life of 3 to 6 hours, that same dose can delay sleep onset, reduce restorative slow-wave sleep, and fragment total sleep time.[266]

Caffeine also delays circadian phase, further misaligning internal clocks already off-kilter.[266]

The problem isn't caffeine. It's timing.

Shift workers often consume caffeine at the wrong times. NHANES data show that while overall intake is similar to daytime workers, night workers tend to drink more caffeine off-shift, when it's most likely to disrupt sleep.[267]

Most follow a general-population rhythm—caffeine in the early morning—even when their "morning" begins after a 12-hour night shift. This is where the gap widens, not between knowledge and caffeine, but between biology and reality.

For many, caffeine isn't used to boost performance. It's used to survive. To get home. To stay awake for a second job or to drive the kids to school. It becomes a last resort, not a strategy.

Mistimed caffeine delays sleep, reduces quality, and builds a debt that compounds into metabolic, cardiovascular, and cognitive risk.[267]

This creates a loop: caffeine for alertness, poor sleep, more fatigue, then more caffeine.

Reactive use builds tolerance, blunts benefits, and increases the risk of dependency.[267] It may also reduce the effectiveness of other countermeasures like melatonin or strategic napping.[267]

Evidence for caffeine's ability to reduce real-world errors or accidents remains limited. It may help alertness, but it does not replace rest.

And yet, guidance is sparse. Few shift-specific caffeine protocols exist. Workers rely on instinct, not evidence.

Best practices suggest stopping caffeine six hours before sleep.[268] Timing it to align with your chronotype, workload, and shift demands. Even better—using tech tools or apps to personalize timing windows.

Caffeine is a tool, but it's a double-edged one.

Used strategically, it sharpens. Used carelessly, it dulls.

Blueprint Supplement Protocol: Caffeine

Category: Targeted Support (Cognitive Stimulation and Circadian-Aligned Alertness)

Form: Naturally occurring stimulant found in brewed coffee, tea, energy drinks, and available as caffeine anhydrous (pill or gum

- Delivery method affects absorption speed—gum and anhydrous forms may produce faster onset compared to brewed forms.

Dose:

- 100–200 mg per serving, with a maximum of 400 mg/day from all sources.
- Lower doses may be sufficient when paired with synergistic compounds (e.g., L-theanine).

Timing:

- Use within the first third of your biological wake cycle, whether that begins at 6:00 a.m. or 6:00 p.m.
- Avoid use within 6–8 hours of intended sleep, to prevent melatonin suppression, sleep latency, and fragmented rest.

Onset:

- Alertness effects begin within 15–30 minutes, with peak impact at ~60 minutes.
- Variability exists based on metabolism, food intake, and habitual use.

Duration:

- Half-life ranges from 3–6 hours, but may be prolonged in slow metabolizers or individuals taking oral contraceptives.

Pairing:

- Combine with L-theanine (100–200 mg) for smoothed focus and reduced jitteriness.

- Avoid concurrent use with alcohol, high-dose nicotine, or late-shift energy drinks, which may overstimulate or disrupt sleep recovery.

Timing Coffee for Longevity and Resilience

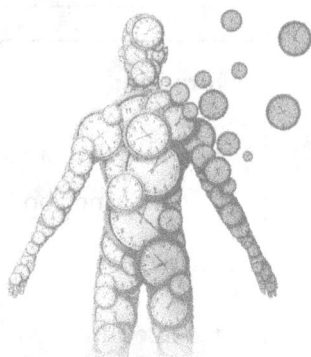

Coffee is not just caffeine. It's a complex biochemical elixir, packed with over a thousand compounds—antioxidants, polyphenols, diterpenes, and more—each with the potential to influence inflammation, metabolism, and cellular aging.[269]

Some of these compounds, like chlorogenic acid, may reduce oxidative stress and improve vascular function, while others, like cafestol in unfiltered brews, may increase LDL cholesterol.[269]

Caffeine may be the headliner, but the supporting cast of bioactive molecules carries weight of its own.

And for shift workers, the benefits, or the risks, depend on more than what's in the cup.

It's about when you drink it.

Because timing, not just content, determines whether coffee sharpens your edge, or blunts your recovery.

Coffee deserves its own chapter, apart from caffeine, because its impact extends far beyond wakefulness. It is one of the most consumed beverages globally and one of the most studied in relation to chronic disease and mortality. Most long-term studies consistently associate moderate coffee consumption, around three to five cups per day, with reduced risk of Type 2 diabetes, cardiovascular disease (CVD), and all-cause mortality.[270] In fact, the 2015–2020 U.S. Dietary Guidelines included moderate coffee intake as part of a healthy eating pattern.[271]

A 2021 study published in *Nutrients* found that moderate habitual coffee consumption was associated with up to a 28% reduction in all-cause mortality, particularly when intake was between 2 and 4 cups per day.[272]

Some benefits, like polyphenol activity, may extend to decaf—but without the stimulant properties, timing becomes less critical.

But beneath the headline lies a murkier reality. The effects of heavy coffee consumption (greater than five cups daily) remain controversial, and a host of modifying variables, from genetics to additives to brew method, may influence outcomes. Researchers have tried to tease out whether health risks or benefits are influenced by decaf status, caffeine metabolism genes, added sugars, or how the coffee is brewed. So far, no consistent pattern has emerged.

But while variables like genetics and brew method remain inconclusive, one factor is gaining clarity: circadian timing.

Recent research suggests that *when* you consume coffee may shape its physiological impact as much as *how much* you consume. Just as meal timing influences metabolism and fat storage, coffee timing may interact with the body's circadian biology, affecting everything from inflammation to cardiovascular health.[272]

This chapter doesn't ask if coffee is "good" or "bad." That binary is outdated. Instead, the question is when, and whether you use coffee for resilience, or let it erode recovery.

And for shift workers, who live outside the boundaries of the traditional solar clock, the timing question becomes even more important.

For the night shift worker, coffee is more than a ritual—it's a decision with biological consequences. The timing of your cup can tilt the balance between resilience and erosion. While caffeine has long been used to battle fatigue, the science now tells us it's not just about drinking coffee—it's about drinking it in harmony with your internal rhythm.

The data are clear: the greatest protective effects on heart health and longevity are seen when coffee is consumed during the *biological morning*, the early part of your wake cycle, not necessarily the time on the clock.[272] Whether you rise at 6 a.m. or 6 p.m., the first 2 to 4 hours after waking is when your body is best equipped to metabolize caffeine, sync with its stimulant effects, and harness its anti-inflammatory benefits. After that window, coffee's upside begins to wane. Drinking it too late, especially near your intended sleep period, disrupts melatonin release, fragments sleep, and initiates a cascade of rhythmic disruptions that may erase its cardiovascular gains.

Anchor coffee to the first third of your wake cycle, taper early, and protect your rest.

Treat coffee as a morning medicine, not an all-night crutch. Used wisely, it becomes a tool for resilience, not dependence, a stimulant transformed into a strategy for longevity.

Drink it early. Drink it intentionally. Let biology, not the breakroom clock, be your guide. In that choice, you reclaim resilience in a schedule designed to take it from you.

Blueprint Supplement Protocol: Coffee

Category: Targeted Stimulant Support

Form: Brewed black coffee (filter or French press preferred). Minimize added sugars and artificial creamers to preserve metabolic benefits.

Dose: 1–3 cups (8 oz each) per 24-hour period is considered moderate and effective for most shift-working adults.

Timing: Consume within the first 2–4 hours of your biological wake cycle, whether that's 6:00 a.m. or 6:00 p.m.

- Avoid intake within 6 hours of intended sleep, as even small doses suppress melatonin and disrupt circadian repair.

Onset: Alertness effects begin within 15–45 minutes; peak plasma concentration at ~60 minutes.

Duration: Caffeine's half-life is 5–7 hours, prolonged in women on oral contraceptives and those with CYP1A2 polymorphisms.

Pairing: Combine with L-theanine (100–200 mg) to buffer overstimulation, reduce jitteriness, and preserve focus.

- Avoid combining with energy drinks or high-dose caffeine supplements, especially late in shift blocks or back-to-back nights.

Calm Without Compromise

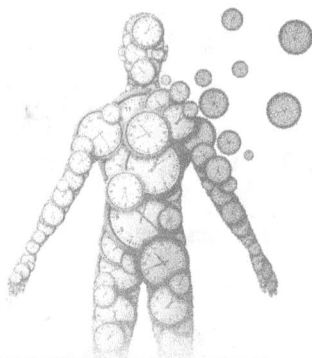

It's 1:00 a.m., and your brain won't stop. You're not fully awake, but not winding down either. Too tired to think. Too wired to rest.

You don't need a sedative.

You need a signal, a way to recalibrate your brain without shutting it off.

Think of it like dimming the lights rather than flipping the switch. This is where L-theanine comes in—not to sedate, but to smooth the edges. Unlike amino acids like leucine or glutamine that support muscle or metabolism, L-theanine operates within the circuits of mood, sleep, and focus.[273]

L-theanine works like a moderator in a tense debate, calming overactive neural circuits, amplifying GABA, and restoring balance between excitatory and inhibitory signals.

Not a tranquilizer. A recalibrator.

L-theanine, an amino acid found in green tea, has emerged as a mild yet effective agent for supporting mental health under conditions of chronic stress and cognitive strain.[274]

L-theanine shares structural similarity with L-glutamic acid and binds to glutamate receptors, modulating neural activity by influencing NMDA receptor activation and shifting the balance between excitation and inhibition. [274]

Through these receptor interactions, L-theanine influences broader neurotransmitter systems—serotonin, dopamine, and GABA—key regulators of mood, stress response, and cognitive function.[275]

In preclinical studies, L-theanine has demonstrated neuroprotective, antidepressant, anxiolytic, and cognitive-enhancing effects, often associated with increased hippocampal BDNF expression and improved synaptic plasticity. [276]

In a randomized, double-blind, placebo-controlled crossover trial, four weeks of 200 mg L-theanine supplementation at night reduced self-reported symptoms of depression, anxiety, and poor sleep quality in adults with subclinical distress.[277]

Most studies use 200 mg at night for sleep support, though doses up to 500 mg daily appear safe and well-tolerated.[277]

L-theanine is classified as Generally Recognized as Safe (GRAS) by the FDA at doses up to 250 mg per day, though most healthy individuals can tolerate up to 500 mg daily without adverse effects.[278]

Its effects are quiet, but they are targeted.

Changes were most pronounced in individuals with lower baseline functioning, suggesting L-theanine is most impactful when stress or cognitive strain is present.[277]

Cognitive performance in verbal fluency and executive function also improved, supporting earlier findings from animal and human studies. [277]

Unlike sedatives or stimulants, L-theanine stabilizes rather than suppresses brain activity, sharpening focus while promoting calm, without impairment or dependence.

Support, not sedation.

Acute use may transiently lower cortisol and enhance immune response, particularly in acutely stressed individuals.[277]

Chronic use may yield broader psychotropic benefits, enhancing stress resilience, cognitive control, and circadian flexibility.[277]

For the night nurse who just finished a code, the EMT whose shift doesn't end when the lights turn off, the parent working nights and waking up early for school drop-off, L-theanine may offer a quiet, daily dose of balance.

It won't change your schedule.

But it may help you meet it, with clarity and calm.

In the broader toolkit of circadian and cognitive resilience, L-theanine stands out as a subtle modulator, realigning mind and mood through the quiet chemistry of neural balance.

Blueprint Supplement Protocol: L-Theanine

Category: Targeted Support (Stress Modulation and Cognitive Calm)

Form: Naturally occurring amino acid, typically sourced from green tea extract; available in capsules or powder form.

- Look for high-purity L-theanine (not racemic or blended forms) for consistent clinical effects.

Dosing:

- 100–200 mg as needed based on stress levels or stimulant use.

- 200 mg nightly may support relaxation, mood regulation, and pre-sleep wind-down over time.

Timing:

- Evening: Take 30–60 minutes before sleep to promote calm without sedation.

- Shift-start: Take 100 mg with caffeine to reduce jitteriness and promote a state of focused calm.

Onset:

- Calming effects begin within 30–60 minutes of ingestion.

- Sleep and mood improvements may accumulate over 1–4 weeks with regular use.

Pairing:

- Combine with magnesium glycinate, apigenin, or glycine for enhanced parasympathetic tone and sleep depth.

- Pair with caffeine during night shifts to sharpen focus while buffering sympathetic overstimulation.

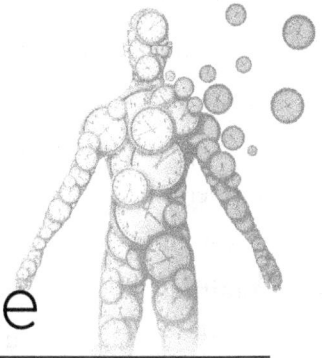

Fuel Without Force

You're not burned out, exactly. But you've lost momentum.

Focus fades. Small tasks feel heavy. You're not depressed, but you're not at baseline either.

ALCAR lives in that middle space. Not a fix-all, but a fueler. Not a stimulant, but a signal—for clarity, energy, and cellular resilience from the inside out. Think of ALCAR like jumper cables, not flooding your system with charge, but restoring the ability to spark

Acetyl-L-carnitine (ALCAR), an acetylated form of L-carnitine, occupies a unique intersection of metabolic regulation and neurochemical modulation relevant to shift workers and individuals exposed to chronic physiological or psychological stress.[279]

It fuels, but doesn't overstimulate.

Known for its role in mitochondrial energy metabolism, facilitating fatty acid transport and buffering acetyl-CoA levels, ALCAR also exerts profound influence on neural plasticity, monoaminergic signaling, and stress resilience.[279]

Research in animal models has demonstrated that short-term ALCAR administration enhances dopamine and serotonin output in the nucleus accumbens, a brain region central to motivation and reward.[280]

Unlike traditional antidepressants, ALCAR enhances dopamine and serotonin within days, without building tolerance, offering rapid but non-sedating neuroadaptation under stress. ALCAR is not a traditional antidepressant or stimulant—it's a calibrator, offering subtle restoration without forceful intervention.[281]

For individuals with diagnosed mood disorders, ALCAR is best seen as an adjunct, not a replacement, for clinically guided treatment.

This suggests that ALCAR may act more as a neuroadaptive modulator than a full-spectrum antidepressant.[281]

ALCAR influences neuronal plasticity through NMDA receptor–dependent pathways and 5-HT1A receptor activation.[281]

Its capacity to increase levels of brain-derived neurotrophic factors, modulate monoamine turnover, and buffer mitochondrial function may underpin its broad but subtle effects on mood, cognition, and stress recovery.

Human studies support its use in age-related cognitive decline, mild depressive symptoms, and neurodegenerative disorders, though its efficacy in major depressive disorder remains inconclusive and may be population specific.[281]

Most human studies use 500–2,000 mg daily, often divided into two doses.

From a pharmacokinetic standpoint, ALCAR's central nervous system effects remain complex.

Despite limited blood-brain barrier penetration, repeated use appears to create cumulative central effects, likely explaining its impact on cognition and stress resilience.[282]

It doesn't force change. It enables capacity.

The compound supports energy metabolism and neuro-transmission, enhancing physical performance, learning capacity, and neuroendocrine feedback in aging or impaired metabolic individuals.

In the context of shift work, where neurochemical imbalances, fatigue, and circadian misalignment are common, ALCAR offers an intriguing adjunct.

Its ability to elevate dopamine and serotonin without sedative or stimulant effects positions it as a potential modulator of alertness, motivation, and emotional stability. [282]

ALCAR's neurochemical enhancements, while robust in acute stress scenarios, do not appear sufficient to reverse chronic behavioral deficits induced by long-term stress, as seen in classical depression models.[283]

It is not a drug of forceful intervention, but of physiological calibration, one that may help readjust energy metabolism and neural signaling in systems strained by irregular sleep, stress, and biological misalignment.

Subtle, not shallow. Real, but quiet.

For the exhausted, but not yet burned out.

For the distracted, but still trying.

For those navigating cognitive slippage under pressure, ALCAR may help hold the line.

It won't energize like caffeine or lift like SSRIs. But it can protect, sustain, and recalibrate the neural systems behind your resilience.

Blueprint Supplement Protocol:
Acetyl-L-Carnitine (ALCAR)

Category: Targeted Support (Cognitive Activation and Mitochondrial Function)

Form: Acetylated amino acid derivative, available in capsule or powder form.

- The ALCAR form is preferred over plain L-carnitine for its neurocognitive and blood–brain barrier permeability advantages.

Dosing:

- Typical range: 500–2,000 mg/day.
- Start with 500–1,000 mg and titrate based on mental fatigue, cognitive load, and tolerance.

Timing:

- Take in the morning or at shift start to enhance focus, motivation, and cellular energy.
- Avoid use within 6–8 hours of intended sleep, as it may produce mild alerting effects in sensitive individuals.

Onset:

- Subjective cognitive enhancements (clarity, stamina, mental drive) often emerge within 7–10 days.
- Deeper mitochondrial and neuroprotective effects build over 4–6 weeks of regular use.

Pairing:

- Combine with CoQ10 or PQQ for mitochondrial synergy and energy metabolism.

- Stack with omega-3 fatty acids or CDP-choline to support neurotransmitter synthesis and cognitive resilience, especially in high-demand shift environments.

Fueling The Fatigued Brain

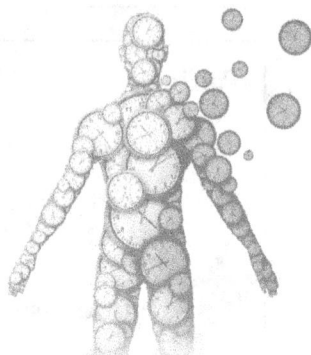

You've been awake for 18 hours. The charting is done, but your brain feels scrambled.

Your shift is over, but now comes the hardest part: the drive home. This is when the fatigue hits. And this is where creatine might matter most.

Creatine stands among the most researched and validated dietary supplements in modern science.[284,285] With over 1,000 peer-reviewed studies supporting its safety and efficacy, creatine has earned a reputation not only as an effective ergogenic aid, enhancing athletic performance, but also for its emerging role in brain health, fatigue resistance, and cellular energy support.[284]

For shift workers battling persistent fatigue and sleep deprivation, creatine, long associated with muscle performance, may offer unexpected benefits for the night shift brain. Unlike caffeine or modafinil, creatine doesn't mask fatigue; it supports your brain's own recovery strategy.

Creatine monohydrate, synthesized in the body and found in meat and fish, functions as a rapid energy reserve by helping regenerate adenosine triphosphate (ATP), the body's cellular fuel.[284] Creatine steps in like auxiliary power during blackout hours—quiet, steady, reliable.

While 95% of the body's creatine resides in skeletal muscle, a small but crucial portion supports brain metabolism.[284]

In the context of shift work, where cognitive demand rises while rest falters, this energy-buffering role becomes more relevant. While these insights began in neurodegenerative disease research, their relevance extends directly to the cognitive strain of shift work.

Creatine is gaining recognition as a potential neuroprotectant under conditions common to shift workers—chronic stress, sleep loss, and circadian disruption.[286]

The brain runs on energy. Creatine supports it by rapidly regenerating ATP, ensuring localized fuel when demand spikes. Research shows creatine may improve cognitive performance under sleep-restricted conditions, enhancing reaction time, memory, and focus.[286]

It protects mitochondria. Reduces oxidative stress. And preserves energy balance during metabolic strain.[286]

In animal studies, creatine has shown neuroprotective effects in Parkinson's and Huntington's disease, acting via membrane stabilization and antioxidant activity.[287]

For night shift workers, creatine may buffer cognitive decline, support mood, and reduce mental fatigue.[287]

A daily dose of 3–5 grams of creatine monohydrate is safe, effective, and requires no cycling.[288]

Creatine is not a stimulant. Its effects are cumulative, not acute. That makes it ideal for long-term support.

During sleep deprivation, the brain's energy systems falter. ATP declines. Mental performance erodes.

Creatine helps refill the tank, restoring ATP and stabilizing function.

In high-demand conditions, single high doses (0.35 g/kg) can improve brain pH, boost executive function, and preserve short-term memory within hours, effects that peak at four hours and last up to nine.[287]

That response depends on demand. When the brain is strained, and creatine is available, it responds.

New data challenge the belief that brain creatine requires weeks to build.[288] Under duress, uptake may increase via altered transporter activity.

This opens a new pathway for performance preservation. Moderate daily doses (0.1 g/kg) or higher doses before long shifts may buffer decline.[289]

Timing matters. Take creatine with your first meal, or with your pre-shift meal, so it's available during the window of peak cognitive demand.[288]

Creatine is not a bypass for rest—it's a contextual tool, most valuable under fatigue and circadian strain.

Open questions remain. Long-term safety. Caffeine interactions. Ideal dosing windows.

Still, for the fatigued brain, creatine is a compelling candidate. Used wisely, it may reduce risk during post-shift tasks and improve performance overnight.

For shift workers, creatine isn't about building strength—it's about preserving clarity, protecting safety, and sustaining resilience when recovery has to wait.

Important Note: Creatine, as discussed in this chapter, should be used contextually—specifically within the framework of shift work, sleep deprivation, and circadian misalignment. Always consult healthcare providers before beginning supplementation.

Some users experience mild GI side effects, often from high doses, low hydration, or taking it on an empty stomach. Symptoms include bloating, cramps, or nausea.[290]

Take creatine with food and stay hydrated to enhance absorption and maximize effectiveness. Micronized creatine may reduce GI issues by improving solubility.[290]

Blueprint Supplement Protocol:

Creatine Monohydrate

Category: Targeted Support (Cognitive Endurance and Cellular Energy)

Form: Use micronized creatine monohydrate for optimal solubility and gastrointestinal tolerance.

- For highest purity and third-party testing, choose Creapure®, a pharmaceutical-grade creatine produced in Germany and widely regarded as the gold standard.

Dosing:

- Maintenance: 5–10 g/day to support ATP regeneration, neuroprotection, and baseline cognitive resilience.

- Acute cognitive stress (e.g., extended shifts, sleep deprivation): up to 0.1–0.35 g/kg body weight, taken prior to or during a demanding shift.

Timing:

- For general resilience: take with the first meal of your wake cycle (day or night).

- For shift-specific demands: dose at the start of your night shift to fuel alertness and reduce cognitive decline during extended hours.

Onset:

- Acute mental performance benefits may begin within 2–4 hours in high-demand settings.

- Neurometabolic saturation occurs after 1–2 weeks of daily use.

Pairing:

- Combine with omega-3 fatty acids to enhance mitochondrial synergy and cognitive stamina.

- Stack with CoQ10 or PQQ during high-fatigue rotations to support energy system restoration and cellular resilience.

The Mitochondrial Recalibrator

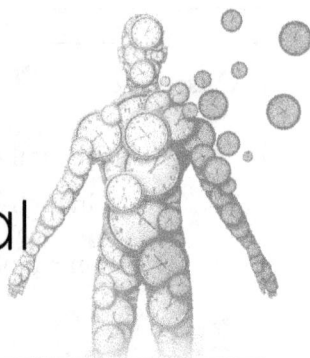

You wake up tired. Not just sleepy—fatigued at the cellular level. Your muscles lag. Your focus drifts. Your body burns fuel inefficiently, like the engine's on, but sputtering. Third night shift in a row. Sleep debt climbing. This is when your mitochondria need backup.

This isn't about motivation. It's about mitochondria. And that's where PQQ comes in.

Pyrroloquinoline quinone (PQQ) is an unassuming nutrient found in vegetables, fruit, even human breast milk.[291]

Yet beneath its dietary ubiquity lies a molecule of profound biological influence, one that modulates mitochondrial performance, antioxidant defense, and cellular resilience under stress.

Shift workers burn through energy. PQQ helps protect and power your cells.

Not through stimulation. Not through sedation. But by enhancing mitochondrial function.

While studied in animal models, recent human trials now affirm that PQQ, as mnemoPQQ®, enhances both muscle strength and functional capacity.[292]

In just 12 weeks, healthy adults taking PQQ showed measurable gains in lower-limb strength, grip force, walking endurance, and mobility tests like the Timed Up and Go (TUG), proof that cellular protection translates into real-world resilience.[293]

These findings align with mechanistic evidence showing that PQQ activates PGC-1α and SIRT1, key regulators of mitochondrial biogenesis and metabolic resilience.[293]

At the cellular level, PQQ prevents oxidative stress-induced mitochondrial dysfunction by preserving structural integrity, respiratory capacity, and redox homeostasis.[293]

In auditory cells exposed to hydrogen peroxide, a model for oxidative damage and cellular senescence, PQQ restored mitochondrial dynamics, supported ATP production, and normalized metabolic signaling through SIRT1/PGC-1 pathways.[294]

This restoration was not superficial.

PQQ improved both mitochondrial fusion and network connectivity, offering protection where aging, stress, or disruption might otherwise erode function.[292]

Across tissues, from skeletal muscle to neurons to systemic metabolism, the theme is consistent: PQQ preserves function under strain.

In skeletal muscle, it suppresses protein degradation pathways activated by inflammation and ROS.[292]

In neurons, it preserves bioenergetics and combats glutamate-induced toxicity. [292]

In systemic physiology, it promotes NAD+ availability and sirtuin activity, an axis increasingly recognized for its role in longevity and cellular efficiency.

Unlike nutrients that exert brute-force effects, PQQ's impact is subtle, cumulative, and systems-oriented.

It facilitates, not dictates, biological recalibration.

It neither sedates nor overstimulates, but rather restores coherence in those drifting from balance.

For shift workers navigating persistent fatigue, disrupted circadian rhythms, and oxidative stress, PQQ offers a targeted, non-stimulating strategy to restore cellular efficiency and resilience.

Its role in enhancing mitochondrial health and preserving bioenergetic function makes it a valuable adjunct to lifestyle protocols aimed at buffering the physiological toll of shift work.

Incorporating PQQ through a high-quality supplement, such as mnemoPQQ®, may support muscular endurance, cognitive clarity, and metabolic balance without interfering with sleep-wake dynamics.[292]

Shift work demands output without offering recovery.

PQQ doesn't offer a shortcut—it offers restoration.

For the exhausted, not the lazy. For the resilient, not the reckless.

This isn't a supplement for stimulation. It's a strategy for stability.

And for shift workers, PQQ isn't about creating more energy—it's about preserving the energy you can't afford to lose.

Blueprint Supplement Protocol:
Pyrroloquinoline Quinone (PQQ)

Category: Targeted Support (Mitochondrial Resilience and Cognitive Stamina)

Form: Redox-active micronutrient available as PQQ disodium salt or proprietary forms like mnemoPQQ®, which may offer enhanced absorption and bioavailability.

- PQQ is not synthesized by the human body and must be obtained through diet or supplementation.

Dosing:

- Standard: 10–20 mg/day for cognitive and mitochondrial support.

- Higher doses (≥20 mg/day) may benefit those experiencing chronic fatigue, cognitive overload, or extended shift blocks.

Timing:

- Take in the morning or at shift start to support mitochondrial activation, alertness, and neuroprotection.

- Avoid taking close to sleep; increased energy metabolism may interfere with wind-down in sensitive users.

Onset:

- Subjective benefits such as increased stamina, mental clarity, and reduced brain fog may appear within 1–2 weeks.

- Structural mitochondrial gains and improved cellular resilience typically accrue over 4–8 weeks of consistent use.

Pairing:

- Combine with CoQ10 for enhanced bioenergetic synergy.

- Stack with magnesium, N-acetylcysteine (NAC), or omega-3s for antioxidant buffering, inflammation reduction, and redox balance, especially valuable in high-stress or night-shift rotations.

Repair From The Inside Out

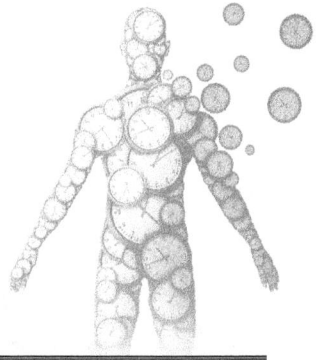

You slept, but you didn't recover. Your body feels inflamed. Fogged. Off-balance. Not because you didn't sleep, but because your sleep didn't repair.

A paramedic wakes after four hours of post-shift sleep—fog thick, joints stiff, motivation gone. It doesn't feel like burnout. It feels like biology, driven by oxidative stress.

This isn't just fatigue—it's cellular fatigue, driven by a buildup of oxidative byproducts that normal sleep can't fully clear.

And N-acetylcysteine (NAC) doesn't sedate—it restores. At the cellular level. Where recovery begins.

Unlike melatonin, which sets the clock, or caffeine, which masks fatigue, NAC clears the oxidative load that fogs the system.

NAC acts as a therapeutic antioxidant, but its most meaningful role may lie in restoring biological balance in individuals under chronic physiological strain, such as shift workers.[295]

Functioning as a precursor to glutathione, NAC enhances the body's capacity to buffer oxidative stress, modulate inflammation, and restore cellular homeostasis.[295]

But its clinical value extends beyond the biochemistry of detoxification.

Emerging research reveals that NAC impacts neurotransmission, sleep regulation, and mitochondrial resilience, suggesting its utility in conditions marked by circadian disruption and redox imbalance.[295]

In both animal models and human trials, NAC has demonstrated neuroprotective effects by crossing the blood-brain barrier and restoring glutathione levels in central nervous system tissues.[296]

These effects appear important under oxidative load, where depleted glutathione contributes to impaired synaptic function and sleep fragmentation.[297]

Studies have shown that NAC accelerates the onset of non-REM sleep, reduces beta activity during quiet wakefulness, and dissipates accumulated sleep pressure, effects that are both restorative and protective.[297]

From a metabolic standpoint, NAC enhances NADPH availability by fueling the glutathione cycle.[296]

Sleep is a redox-driven process—rest clears oxidative stress, and compounds like NAC support this recovery.

Experimental studies show that NAC reduces EEG markers of sleep pressure and redirects brain metabolism from oxidative to more efficient pathways.[298] And beyond sleep, NAC's effects ripple across multiple systems under stress.

In cardiovascular care, it improves myocardial rescue during acute infarction, enhances nitric oxide signaling, and reduces postoperative arrhythmias.[299]

In neurology, researchers have linked glutathione elevation in individuals with Parkinson's disease and multiple sclerosis to improved mitochondrial function and enhanced cognitive performance.[300]

In psychiatry, NAC's modulation of glutamate transmission and inflammatory signaling has led to its use in mood disorders, schizophrenia, and substance use disorders.[301]

Most relevant for shift workers, NAC's role in sleep physiology is beginning to come into focus.

Beyond its general antioxidant properties, NAC alters sleep architecture and timing in ways that are both measurable and meaningful.

The effects are sex-specific—males and females exhibit divergent responses in EEG dynamics following NAC administration.[302]

These differences underscore the importance of individualized dosing and timing when treating conditions characterized by sleep fragmentation and oxidative burden.

NAC's pharmacological profile is well-characterized.

It is affordable, bioavailable in oral dosing, and well-tolerated.

Most studies use oral doses of 600–1,200 mg daily, often divided, which appear both safe and effective.[295]

Mild gastrointestinal symptoms are the most common side effects, and anaphylactoid reactions to intravenous forms are rare.

Not a bandage. A buffer.

It clears the fog, at the level of cells.

Your sleep can't repair what your system can't detox.

For the shift worker whose sleep is shallow, whose thoughts feel thick, and whose body runs on fumes, NAC is not a sedative—it's a signal. A quiet push toward balance, clarity, and the kind of restorative sleep that sustains resilience in a schedule that won't.

Blueprint Supplement Protocol:

N-Acetylcysteine (NAC)

Category: Targeted Support (Redox Regulation, Sleep Recovery, and Cognitive Resilience)

Form: Available in oral capsules, powders, or effervescent tablets.

- Use pharmaceutical-grade NAC for consistent dosing and absorption.

- Note: NAC has a sulfur-like taste/smell; effervescent formats may improve palatability.

Dosing:

- 600–1,200 mg/day, split into one or two doses based on tolerance and intent (sleep vs daytime support).

- For extended stress or toxic load, consider guided dosing protocols with a licensed provider.

Timing:

- For sleep restoration and glutathione replenishment: take 600 mg 1–2 hours before intended sleep.

- For daytime redox support and cognitive clarity: take early in the shift to support oxidative balance.

Onset:

- Subjective improvements (less brain fog, reduced fatigue) may appear within 7–10 days.

- Deeper mitochondrial support and improvements in sleep architecture build over 2–4 weeks.

Pairing:

- Combine with magnesium or glycine to enhance parasympathetic tone and sleep depth.

- Stack with omega-3s, CoQ10, or PQQ to reinforce mitochondrial efficiency, antioxidant defense, and neuroprotection, especially during high oxidative demand or night-shift recovery.

The Neural Stabilizer

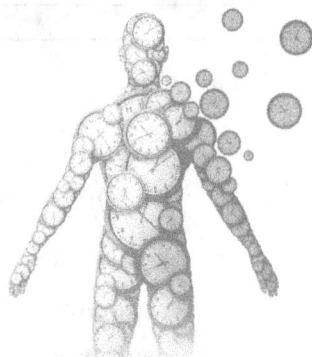

You're alert at 2 a.m., but barely.

Your thoughts lag behind your actions. Cortisol surges. Patience frays. And sleep, when it finally comes, feels like a failed reboot. This isn't just tiredness. It's neural instability.

And that's where phosphatidylserine begins to matter.

For shift workers navigating chronic fatigue, fragmented sleep, and cognitive strain, phosphatidylserine (PS) offers more than just cellular support: it acts as a neurobiological stabilizer, helping the brain recalibrate under pressure.

A structural phospholipid concentrated in brain cell membranes, PS plays a critical role in neurotransmission, stress regulation, and inflammation.[303]

While often overshadowed in mainstream sleep science, PS, and its synergistic pairing with omega-3 polyunsaturated fatty acids (PUFAs), emerges as a quiet agent of circadian resilience.[304]

Phosphatidylserine supports neuronal signaling, fuels cellular energy production, and drives the synthesis of key neurotransmitters: acetylcholine, dopamine, norepinephrine, and serotonin.[303]

These pathways intersect with those governing mood, cognition, and sleep.

In animal models with Parkinsonian traits and disrupted sleep, PS supplementation restored brain levels of PS and normalized circadian sleep patterns.[305]

PS also resensitizes cortisol receptors that have become desensitized by chronic stress exposure, allowing more effective regulation of the HPA axis.[303]

This action facilitates a return to homeostasis, lowering circulating cortisol levels and promoting deeper, more restorative sleep.

Phosphatidylserine supports serotonin synthesis and transmission, both crucial for stabilizing mood and improving sleep architecture.[303]

For shift workers battling chronic stress and circadian misalignment, these effects translate into better emotional regulation, deeper sleep, and greater resilience on and off the job.

From a neuroprotective perspective, PS reduces pro-inflammatory cytokines such as TNF-α and IL-1β and increases anti-inflammatory markers like TGF-β.[305]

This dual action, reducing inflammation while stabilizing cellular membranes, may explain PS's benefits across a range of neurodegenerative and neuropsychiatric conditions, including Alzheimer's, Parkinson's, depression, ADHD, and stroke.[305]

But its relevance isn't limited to disease—these same mechanisms apply directly to the chronic stress and misalignment faced by shift workers.

In older adults, a 12-week protocol combining PS and omega-3 PUFAs taken three times daily lowers baseline cortisol levels and reestablishes circadian rhythm patterns in salivary cortisol.[306]

These changes coincide with measurable symptom improvement in individuals with major depression.

Phosphatidylserine, alone or with omega-3s, improves sleep quality and supports cognitive function.[306]

Due to concerns about prion transmission from bovine-derived products, plant-based preparations, like those from soybeans or sunflowers, are now preferred.[307]

Supplementation periods of 6 to 15 weeks have improved short-term memory and cognitive clarity in older adults with memory complaints.[308]

For shift workers, the implications are profound.

Sleep loss. Elevated cortisol. Cognitive wear.

PS offers a nutritional countermeasure, supporting brain health not through stimulation, but through repair.

It doesn't override exhaustion. It recalibrates.

When taken with omega-3s, PS helps restore circadian signals, reduce neuroinflammation, and preserve mental clarity.

Most studies suggest 300–800 mg daily, taken with meals and divided into two or three doses, though shift-specific protocols are still lacking.[303]

In a body asked to push against time, PS doesn't push back. It steadies. It softens the blow of stress and restores rhythms that fatigue unravels.

Blueprint Supplement Protocol:
Phosphatidylserine (PS)

Category: Targeted Support (Cortisol Modulation, Cognitive Clarity, and Circadian Stabilization)

Form: A structural phospholipid found in neuronal membranes.

- Opt for plant-derived sources (soy or sunflower) for optimal purity, consistency, and safety profile.

Dosing:

- 300–800 mg/day, divided into 2–3 doses.

- Individual response varies—start low and titrate based on stress load, mood, and sleep response.

Timing:

- Take with fat-containing meals to support absorption and transport across the blood–brain barrier.

- For cortisol regulation and sleep preparation, schedule the final dose in the early evening or during post-shift wind-down.

Onset:

- Cognitive and mood improvements typically appear within 2–4 weeks.

- Cortisol stabilization and circadian entrainment may require 6–12 weeks of consistent use in shift workers with chronic HPA axis dysregulation.

Pairing:

- Combine with omega-3 fatty acids (EPA/DHA) to boost neuroprotective and circadian alignment effects.

- Stack with magnesium or L-theanine for deeper stress buffering and pre-sleep parasympathetic activation.

Fueling The Fatigued Cell

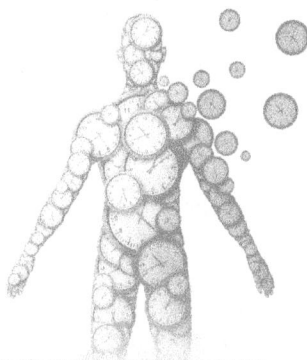

By the time your fourth night shift hits, the fatigue is no longer just tiredness—it's inside your cells. You're not sleepy. You're running inefficiently. CoQ10 works where stimulants fail, deep within your mitochondria, where energy is actually made.

In the battle against shift work–related fatigue, where sleep loss and cognitive strain are daily realities, Coenzyme Q10 (CoQ10) offers a compelling, evidence-backed intervention.

Known primarily for its role in ATP and mitochondrial energy production as well as antioxidant defense, CoQ10 emerges as a biological safeguard in systems taxed by irregular hours and chronic exhaustion.[309]

It's not a stimulant. It's not a mask. It's a mechanism.

This fat-soluble, vitamin-like compound plays a vital role in ATP production, transferring electrons within the mitochondrial respiratory chain while protecting mitochondrial membranes and cellular DNA from oxidative damage.[310]

For shift workers, it may provide not just metabolic reinforcement, but resilience at the cellular level.

A randomized, double-blind, placebo-controlled trial demonstrated the utility of CoQ10 in frontline healthcare. Nurses who took 200 mg of CoQ10 daily for four weeks reported greater energy and better sleep quality compared to those who received a placebo.[311]

Over half of participating nurses met the threshold for clinical fatigue, a condition tied to the number of shifts worked per month.

Though systemic solutions like reduced workloads often remain out of reach in clinical settings, CoQ10 supplementation has proven to be a safe and practical strategy for mitigating fatigue under real-world conditions.

And while its most immediate benefits are felt in fatigue, its long-term value lies in slowing the cellular wear-and-tear that shift work accelerates.[311]

Its unique bioenergetic and antioxidant functions help buffer mitochondrial decline, reduce oxidative stress, and protect DNA integrity, factors tied to neurodegeneration and cellular aging.

CoQ10 enrichment in platelets and white blood cells increases antioxidant capacity and lowers DNA damage markers.[311]

These intracellular effects may take weeks to develop, but they can persist even after supplementation ends.

Unlike stimulants, CoQ10 doesn't force energy.

It preserves it.

Its distribution is uneven across tissues and relies on endogenous synthesis.

This makes supplementation relevant in high-demand or deficiency states.

Uptake into mitochondria-rich cells like platelets and leukocytes depends on physiological need and mitochondrial demand.

For shift workers, whose schedules disrupt not only circadian rhythm but also mitochondrial and neurochemical homeostasis, CoQ10 offers targeted support.

It helps restore the systems that fatigue erodes.

Most studies use 100–300 mg daily, taken with a fat-containing meal to maximize absorption; plasma levels peak within 6–8 hours.[309]

In a workforce forced to operate beyond its biological blueprint, CoQ10 supports cellular stability.

Not by stimulating.

By restoring balance.

In a body that's chronically overdrawn, CoQ10 is cellular credit. Not fast cash like caffeine. Not a mask. A mechanism. Quietly restoring resilience, one mitochondrion at a time.

Blueprint Supplement Protocol:
Coenzyme Q10 (CoQ10)

Category: Targeted Support (Mitochondrial Energy, Fatigue Resistance, and Cellular Protection)

Form: A fat-soluble quinone compound, available in two primary forms:

- Ubiquinone (oxidized) – widely available and cost-effective.

- Ubiquinol (reduced) – more bioavailable, often preferred for older adults or individuals with high oxidative stress.

Dosing:

- Typical range: 100–300 mg/day.

- Ubiquinol may require lower dosing (100–200 mg) due to enhanced absorption and higher plasma retention.

Timing:

- Take with a fat-containing meal, ideally with your largest meal or at shift start to support energy production and antioxidant defense throughout the waking period.

Onset:

- Plasma levels peak 6–8 hours after ingestion.

- Mitochondrial benefits—such as improved endurance, reduced fatigue, and enhanced cognitive function—typically emerge within 2–4 weeks of consistent use.

Pairing:

- Combine with magnesium and omega-3 fatty acids to enhance ATP synthesis and neurovascular stability.

- Stack with PQQ to promote mitochondrial biogenesis, especially during high-demand shifts or chronic fatigue states.

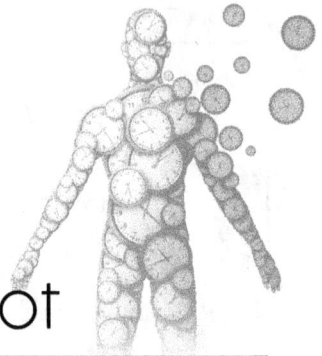

The Resilience Root

It's 4:15 a.m. in the surgical ICU. A resident leans against the med cart, charting with one hand, sipping cold coffee with the other. The buzz from the caffeine is gone. What remains is something heavier: an ache behind the eyes, a mind that won't focus, and a heart that won't stop racing.

They're not sleepy.

They're scrambled.

It's their second 24-hour call in four days, and everything feels like it's happening through a fog. The instinct is to push harder. But what their system needs isn't more stimulation—it's recovery. That's where rhodiola rosea enters the conversation.

For centuries, communities in the harsh climates of Siberia and the Arctic turned to rhodiola rosea, known as "golden root", to boost stamina, fight fatigue, and restore vitality in unforgiving environments.[312]

For modern shift workers living under a different form of biological stress, this adaptogen may offer a resilient ally.

Rhodiola's reputation stems not just from tradition, but from emerging evidence across multiple domains of health: fatigue, mood, cognition, physical performance, reproductive health, and even cardiovascular function.[312]

As an adaptogen, rhodiola does not target one symptom; it supports systemic balance under stress.

Adaptogens help normalize disrupted physiology, making them relevant for shift workers navigating chronic circadian misalignment.[313]

Rhodiola rosea influences multiple stress-related pathways. It modulates cortisol levels, enhances beta-endorphin activity, and regulates key neurotransmitters, including serotonin and dopamine.[313]

These effects may translate into improved energy, mood stability, and cognitive resilience.

Among the most well-studied benefits of rhodiola rosea is its impact on fatigue.

In clinical trials, rhodiola improved mental performance, attention, and reaction time in individuals exposed to night shift work, academic stress, or burnout.[314]

In physicians working overnight shifts, rhodiola supplementation improved fatigue indices and short-term memory.[314]

In students undergoing examination stress, it enhanced mood stability, reduced the need for sleep, and improved coordination and motivation.

It's not a stimulant. It's a stabilizer.

And in the psychological terrain of shift work, where clarity gives way to volatility, this distinction matters.

Yet like most adaptogens, rhodiola isn't one-size-fits-all. In one trial, student nurses saw no benefit, a reminder that dose matters. While earlier studies used up to 680 mg/day, this trial used just 364 mg/day.[315]

This discrepancy highlights the need for dosage optimization. It also reminds us that adaptogens aren't magic—they're tools. Their success depends on context: the dose, the extract, and the system receiving them.

Rhodiola's effects on mood disorders, mild-to-moderate depression, and anxiety are documented.[314]

It has reduced symptoms of generalized anxiety disorder (GAD), improved sleep, and lowered cortisol awakening response in patients with burnout.[314]

Compared to conventional antidepressants, rhodiola produced fewer side effects and similar clinical improvement.[314]

For shift workers facing psychological fatigue, sleep disruption, and emotional volatility, rhodiola offers low-risk, moderate-reward support.

While rhodiola's cognitive benefits take center stage, its effects go deeper. The cardiovascular system, particularly vulnerable to chronic stress and circadian strain, may also benefit.

Preclinical studies show rhodiola can decrease stress-induced cardiac damage, lower blood pressure, and improve endothelial function.[316]

For shift workers, already at elevated risk of cardiovascular and reproductive disruption, these findings add weight to rhodiola's role as a systemic buffer.

It's subtle. But powerful. Not intensity—resilience.

Rhodiola's antioxidant and cardioprotective benefits may protect long-term cardiovascular health in shift-working populations.[316] But stress doesn't stop at the heart. It reaches deeper, disrupting hormonal rhythms that influence fertility, libido, and reproductive timing.

Reproductive benefits are less studied, but early findings are promising.

Rhodiola may help restore ovulation in women with amenorrhea and improve sexual function in men with erectile dysfunction.[317]

It modulates the hypothalamic–pituitary–gonadal axis, where stress often disrupts fertility.[316,317]

Athletes have long turned to rhodiola for endurance and recovery.

In trials, it improved anaerobic power, reduced perceived exertion, increased antioxidant capacity, and reduced muscle damage.[318]

The same benefits may extend to shift workers who train under fatigue or time constraints.

Not all extracts are created equal.

Therapeutic benefits occur when formulations contain at least 3% rosavins and 1% salidroside.

Results vary depending on standardization, timing, and individual variability in stress response.[318]

Rhodiola rosea stands where ancient tradition meets modern physiology.

It modulates when your system is out of rhythm, and buffers when recovery feels out of reach.

In the architecture of recovery, rhodiola isn't the foundation, but it may be the scaffolding.

For those who perform under pressure, sleep in fragments, and live out of sync, this golden root offers something rare: resilience—accessible, adaptable, and in plant form.

Blueprint Supplement Protocol: Rhodiola rosea

Category: Targeted Support (Stress Resilience, Mental Stamina, and HPA Axis Modulation)

Form: Use a standardized extract containing ≥3% rosavins and ≥1% salidroside, the clinically supported ratio for adaptogenic benefits.

- Ensure third-party testing for potency and purity.

Dosing:

- General support: 200–400 mg/day, taken 30–60 minutes before shift start or during high-stress windows.
- ≤200 mg may be effective for mild fatigue or ongoing maintenance.
- Higher doses (400–680 mg) are often used for cognitive strain, emotional burnout, or sustained overload.

Timing:

- Take in the morning or pre-shift to activate mental performance and stress adaptation.
- Avoid late-day dosing in sensitive individuals, as mild overstimulation may interfere with sleep.

Onset:

- Acute improvements in fatigue and alertness can appear within 1–2 hours.
- Full adaptogenic effects typically develop over 1–2 weeks of regular use.

Pairing:

- Combine with L-theanine for calm, sustained focus without overstimulation.

- Stack with omega-3 fatty acids to reinforce mood stability and HPA axis regulation, especially during shift transitions or recovery periods.

The Root That Adapts and Endures

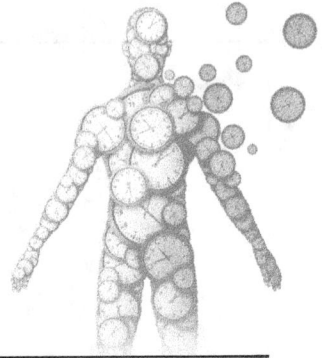

At 8:30 p.m., a nurse checks their vitals for the second time, chest tight, mood flat, thoughts scattered.

Not panic.

Not exhaustion.

Just the steady hum of system-wide strain.

They're not looking for sleep. They're looking for reset.

Somewhere between adrenaline and depletion, their biology forgets what time it is. And every system—hormonal, cognitive, emotional—follows.

In the 24/7 grind of modern labor, where productivity runs on borrowed time, the shift worker becomes a physiological outlier. Amid the wear and tear, another ancient root, ashwagandha (*Withania somnifera*), emerges as a rare botanical constant.

Used for centuries in Ayurvedic medicine, ashwagandha is classified as an adaptogen.[319] Not a stimulant. Not a sedative. But something that normalizes. It helps the body respond to both physical and psychological stress.[319] But what happens when the stressor isn't external, but internal—when time itself is the adversary?

Beyond folklore, the science is catching up.

A 16-week randomized, placebo-controlled trial explored ashwagandha's effects in overweight men aged 40–70 with mild fatigue. Hormone levels, not mood scores, told the real story. Participants taking a standardized extract (Shoden® beads delivering 21 mg of withanolide glycosides) experienced an 18% rise in DHEA-S and a nearly 15% increase in testosterone, without crossing into abnormal levels or triggering adverse effects.[320]

For shift workers, this matters: hormonal erosion happens subtly, long before clinical deficiency is flagged. ashwagandha's ability to nudge these systems back toward balance, without overcorrecting, makes it rare among nonpharmacologic tools.

Cortisol remained unchanged. But DHEA-S, an adrenal marker of physiological resilience, told another tale.[320] And one in five participants in the trial worked shifts or in mines. The relevance to chronically stressed, biologically misaligned workers is impossible to ignore.

Cortisol, testosterone, and melatonin are all governed by circadian rhythm.[321] When that rhythm breaks, hormonal chaos follows, and ashwagandha's ability to stabilize stress hormones and modulate anabolic pathways becomes especially relevant for shift workers.

But intention matters. This is not a casual supplement. It's a tool. Its timing must mirror your reality.

Anchor your dose to the *start* of your biological day, whatever the clock says. For night shift, that's pre-shift. For early risers, that's post-dinner. Let the rhythm of your work define the rhythm of your dose.

For rotating schedules: pair your dose with your circadian pattern, not the time on your watch. Ashwagandha works best when it supports your stress load, not your sleep directly.

It calms, not by forcing rest, but by restoring the signaling systems that make rest possible. It's not a knockout agent. It's a neurological exhale.

Unlike pharmaceutical hormone therapies, ashwagandha operates within physiologic limits. Most studies use daily doses of 120–240 mg standardized extract, typically taken once or twice depending on formulation.[319]

Reviews confirm its tolerability in anxious adults, sleep-disrupted workers, and even infertile men. Dependency is rare. Benefits, cumulative.

Not all formulations deliver. The research is based on Shoden®, a GMP-certified extract with standardized withanolide content.[322] Without this, the benefits may not translate.

Modern shift workers face a unique biology: exhausted but alert, awake when the world sleeps. Ashwagandha doesn't erase the misalignment.

It steadies what time shakes, restoring resilience where exhaustion takes root.

And in a life structured by someone else's schedule, that quiet recalibration may be the most powerful form of resistance.

Let your biology, not your clock, determine your dose.

Blueprint Supplement Protocol:

Ashwagandha (Withania somnifera)

Category: Targeted Support (Stress Adaptation, Hormonal Resilience, and Circadian Modulation)

Form: Root-based adaptogen, ideally in a standardized extract form.

- Evidence-backed formulations include Shoden® (high bioavailability, 21 mg withanolide glycosides) and KSM-66® (full-spectrum root extract with established clinical data).

Dosing:

- Shoden®: 120–240 mg/day for enhanced absorption and low-dose efficacy.

- KSM-66®: 300–600 mg/day, often preferred for generalized stress, cortisol regulation, and physical fatigue.

Timing:

- Night shift workers: take 30–60 minutes before shift start to support energy, calm, and HPA axis regulation.

- Early/morning shift: dose in the early evening to help regulate overnight hormonal recovery.

- Rotating shifts: anchor dosing to your biological rhythm, not the clock—take consistently relative to your internal circadian timing.

Onset:

- Subjective improvements in stress tolerance, anxiety, and energy may emerge within 1–2 weeks.

- Hormonal and adaptogenic benefits (e.g., cortisol modulation, thyroid support) typically accumulate over 8–16 weeks.

Pairing:

- Combine with magnesium or L-theanine for parasympathetic synergy and pre-shift stability.

- Stack with omega-3s or vitamin D3 to support hormonal balance, immune readiness, and long-term circadian adaptation.

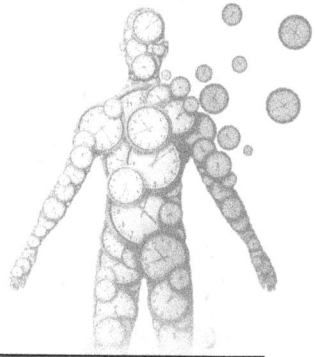

REM Without Rest

At 4:19 a.m., a trauma nurse stares at the computer, blinking harder than usual.

The name is familiar. The weight, the age, the diagnosis—familiar. But charting is delayed. Recognition is slow to surface.

It's not forgetfulness. It's sleep deprivation.

And when REM vanishes, memory loses its tether.

In the misaligned world of shift work, where fragmented sleep and mistimed light exposure clash with biology, REM sleep fractures first. Lost in the absence of natural light and consistent rest, REM sleep may disappear without notice, but its absence leaves a deep physiological trace. And the brain keeps score long after the shift ends.

What's happening here isn't failure—it's physiology. And it starts with the quiet collapse of REM.

This phase of sleep plays a critical role in memory consolidation, emotional regulation, and neuroplasticity.[323] It facilitates long-term potentiation, the foundational process through which the brain encodes new information.

When REM disappears, hippocampal plasticity weakens.[323] Antioxidant defenses drop. Oxidative stress builds in the brain's most memory-critical regions.

But where vulnerability exists, so does opportunity.

Where REM loss destabilizes cognition, CDP-choline intervenes at the molecular level to preserve clarity.

CDP-choline (citicoline), an endogenous compound involved in the synthesis of acetylcholine and phosphatidylcholine, has emerged as a potent neuroprotective agent.[324]

Where REM loss destabilizes cognition, CDP-choline intervenes at the molecular level to preserve clarity.

In animal models deprived of REM sleep for 96 hours, memory deficits appeared, until CDP-choline was introduced.[324] Supplementation restored antioxidant capacity and reversed the decline in pCaMKII expression.[325] A molecular rescue of function.

For shift workers living with chronic REM debt, CDP-choline is more than theory—it's strategy.

Choline supports neurotransmission, membrane repair, and methylation, essential for balanced serotonin, dopamine, and cognitive stability.[326] While foods like eggs and meats offer modest doses, the demands of shift work often exceed dietary supply. And because choline synthesis declines under chronic stress, the gap between what you need and what you get quietly widens.

CDP-choline offers a direct, measurable benefit. It restores cognitive precision, memory stability, and motor coordination lost when REM fractures.

As a precursor to acetylcholine, choline influences reaction time, attention, and neuromotor performance. Rodents deprived of choline show deficits in learning and coordination; supplementation reverses those declines.[327]

Once dismissed as nutritionally non-essential, choline is now recognized as foundational, supporting everything from neurotransmission to liver health.

Despite this, few occupational health strategies incorporate choline. Most focus on hydration, caffeine, or calories. Few address the neurochemical cost of REM fragmentation. But in roles where memory means safety, and clarity can't wait, this omission matters.

CDP-choline fills that gap.

In studies, CDP-choline improved executive function, working memory, and verbal recall, especially in those starting from a place of cognitive fatigue.[327] These effects are most relevant for shift workers in high-risk environments: ICU nurses, paramedics, night-shift operators.

Two primary forms exist: CDP-choline (citicoline) and alpha-GPC. CDP-choline supports memory and neuroprotection.[328] Alpha-GPC may enhance neuromotor control and precision.[328]

Most tolerate choline well. Side effects are rare—mild nausea or headache in some. It pairs synergistically with magnesium, B vitamins, and omega-3s. But consult a clinician if you have bipolar disorder or use cholinergic drugs.

Most studies use 250–500 mg daily, often divided into two doses.[328]

In a world shaped by fragmented sleep and relentless demand, choline is more than a supplement—it's a defense. A biochemical scaffold for resilience.

REM sleep cannot always be reclaimed. But its losses can be mitigated.

In the night-shift world of cortisol spikes and neurological cost, CDP-choline offers something rare: A quiet but powerful promise. That some functions can be repaired. That some clarity can be restored. And that some rhythms, with the right support, can return.

Back at the computer, the nurse recenters. The name comes back. The brain still remembers—when it's given the tools to restore resilience.

Blueprint Supplement Protocol:
CDP-Choline (Citicoline)

Category: Targeted Support (Cognitive Activation, Memory Recovery, and Neurotransmitter Balance)

Form: A water-soluble choline compound, available as CDP-choline (Citicoline) or Alpha-GPC

- CDP-choline supports acetylcholine production, dopaminergic tone, and neuronal membrane repair.

- Alpha-GPC may offer stronger neuromotor and physical performance effects.

Dosing:

- CDP-Choline:

  - 250–500 mg in the morning for general cognitive support.

  - 500–1,000 mg/day, split into two doses, to target REM-related memory recovery or post-shift cognitive fatigue.

- Alpha-GPC: 300–600 mg, taken 30–60 minutes pre-shift, to support reaction time, focus, and neuromotor function.

Timing:

- Take in the morning or at the start of your shift to promote alertness, executive function, and working memory.

- Avoid dosing within 6 hours of sleep, as mild cholinergic stimulation may delay onset in sensitive individuals.

Onset:

- Noticeable improvements in attention, clarity, and verbal fluency may emerge within 1–2 weeks.\

- Deeper neuroplastic benefits, including memory consolidation and REM-linked cognitive recovery, may build over 4–6 weeks of consistent use.

P airing:

- Combine with magnesium, B-complex vitamins, and omega-3s (especially DHA) to optimize cholinergic tone, membrane repair, and neurotransmitter function.

- Ensure adequate hydration, as cholinergic support is sensitive to fluid status and electrolyte balance.

The Plant That Restores Pattern

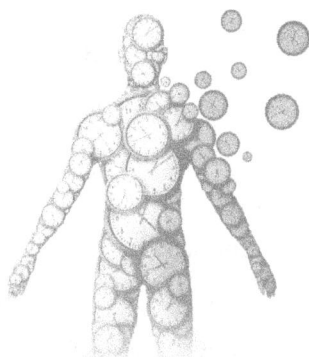

They finish the night shift at 7:30 a.m. and stare at the sunrise—not with awe, but with dread. Sleep should come easily. It doesn't. The body is wired. The thoughts are frayed.

Enter apigenin, not as a sedative, but as a quiet recalibrator. A signal that sleep is safe again.

In a world of artificial lighting, fragmented sleep, and age-accelerating stressors, the need for natural compounds that target both brain health and circadian resilience has never been greater. Melatonin is delayed. Cortisol rises when it should fall. And rest becomes a memory instead of a guarantee.

Apigenin, a flavonoid abundant in chamomile, parsley, celery, and other plant-based foods, has emerged as a promising agent at the intersection of sleep science, neuroprotection, and healthy aging.[329]

Recognized for its calming effects, apigenin exerts mild sedative properties long associated with chamomile tea. But its power runs deeper. It inhibits CD38, a NADase enzyme that depletes cellular NAD+, a molecule central to energy, repair, and longevity.[329]

By preserving NAD+, apigenin enhances mitochondrial performance, reduces inflammation, and boosts brain plasticity.[330]

In animal models, this translates into improved learning, memory, and more stable sleep.[330]

Sleep loss and aging travel the same neurobiological paths—both impair synaptic plasticity, elevate oxidative stress, and destabilize hippocampal networks. Apigenin counters each step.

It also acts on dopamine and monoamine oxidase, improving mood by day and easing the transition into sleep by night. These effects scale with dose and are enhanced through gut metabolism, as the microbiome converts apigenin into even more bioactive compounds.

For shift workers, whose disrupted sleep and diet erode microbial diversity, apigenin helps repair the gut-brain axis. This is botanical circadian therapy.

Its benefits don't stop at the brain. Apigenin improves glucose handling, reduces fat accumulation, and stabilizes cardiovascular function in metabolic models.[330] For shift workers at risk for insulin resistance and inflammation, it offers a wide-spectrum shield.

Human trials of chamomile extract, apigenin's primary source, show improved sleep onset and reduced anxiety, validating what centuries of tradition have observed.[331] While apigenin is one of chamomile's key active compounds, no shift-specific dosing protocols yet exist.

Apigenin isn't just about relaxation. It's about repair.

In shift workers, it targets the damage left by mistimed light, missing REM, and cortisol overload. It doesn't force sedation—it restores rhythm. Its actions are subtle, systemic, and deeply aligned with the biology of rest and resilience.

While many apigenin benefits stem from animal or whole-plant studies, its isolated effects remain under review.

In a world where dawn brings dread, apigenin offers a reminder, not just that rest is possible, but that resilience can be restored.

Blueprint Supplement Protocol: Apigenin

Category: Targeted Support (Sleep Architecture, Circadian Recovery, and Neuro-calming)

Form: A naturally occurring flavonoid found in chamomile, parsley, and celery, available in standardized extracts or capsule form.

- Look for high-purity apigenin with known sourcing to ensure potency and consistency.

Dosing:

- 25–50 mg daily is typical for sleep support and circadian entrainment.

- Higher doses (up to 100 mg/day) may be found in longevity or mitochondrial support stacks, but should be titrated cautiously.

Timing:

- Take 30–60 minutes before intended sleep, especially after night shifts or when preparing for daytime recovery sleep.

- Ideal as part of a pre-sleep wind-down protocol for shift workers.

Onset:

- Calming and GABAergic effects may be noticeable within several days.

- Mitochondrial and circadian-phase benefits typically develop over 2–4 weeks of consistent use.

Pairing:

- Combine with magnesium glycinate, glycine, or L-theanine to enhance GABAergic tone, sleep latency, and overall sleep architecture.

- May be used alongside applied light-blocking strategies (e.g., blue-light filters or blackout curtains) to amplify circadian effects.

Sleep, Repair, and the Brain That Never Clocks Out

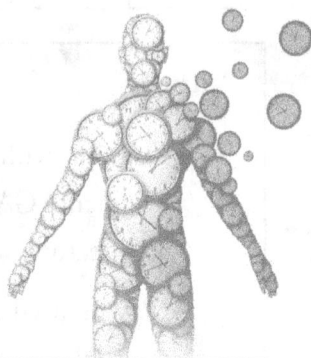

It's 3:00 a.m. again.

The fluorescent lights hum overhead. Their hands are steady, but their memory isn't. There's fog where clarity should be. Fatigue where sharpness used to live.

And tomorrow, they'll do it all again.

But chronic sleep fragmentation doesn't just steal clarity—it accelerates neurobiological aging. It depletes BDNF, erodes synaptic resilience, and raises the long-term risk of neurodegeneration.

An unassuming mushroom, centuries old, and newly relevant.

In a world where sleep is scarce and anxiety abundant, few natural compounds offer the dual therapeutic potential of *Hericium erinaceus*, known as lion's mane mushroom.

Lion's mane, used as both food and medicine, is a neurotrophic fungus that has attracted growing scientific interest for its ability to improve sleep quality, regulate mood, and promote neural regeneration, benefits that resonate with the physiologic burdens of shift work.[332]

Lion's mane doesn't sedate—it rebuilds.

Rich in bioactive compounds such as hericenones and erinacines, this fungus stimulates the production of brain-derived neurotrophic factor and nerve growth factor (NGF), both of which are essential for neuroplasticity, mood regulation, and REM sleep integrity.[333]

In human studies, including a 4-week administration of a standardized extract (Amyloban® 3399), lion's mane was associated with significant reductions in depression, irritability, and fatigue.[334]

Female university students, a population at considerable risk for sleep and mood disorders, reported improvements in sleep quality and general well-being after supplementation.[334]

Preclinical research has deepened this promise.

In animal models subjected to stress-induced sleep deprivation, high-dose lion's mane mycelium (150 mg/kg) reversed disruptions in non-REM (NREM) and REM sleep.[335]

Notably, lion's mane suppressed the pathological REM rebound, a phenomenon where lost REM returns in excess, often fragmented or maladaptive, observed in stressed animals, supporting a healthier distribution of sleep phases.[335] Lion's mane didn't just restore REM, it helped normalize its rhythm.

These effects are dose-dependent: while lower doses showed modest benefits, the 150 mg/kg dose improved both behavioral and neurochemical markers.[336]

The anxiolytic effects of lion's mane are also compelling.

Unlike conventional anxiolytics, lion's mane exerts its effects through the restoration of dopamine levels rather than sedation or serotonin modulation.

At the molecular level, lion's mane crosses the blood-brain barrier and modulates key signaling pathways including BDNF/TrkB/PI3K/Akt/GSK-3 .[336]

Its compounds preserve existing neuronal architecture while promoting the growth of new synapses, an action important in sleep-deprived or stressed brains.

In models of neurodegenerative disease, lion's mane has demonstrated potential in reversing early Alzheimer's-like pathology.[337]

A recent placebo-controlled trial showed cognitive preservation in aging adults who consumed capsules enriched with erinacine A, a bioactive compound found in the mycelium of *Hericium erinaceus*.[337]

These findings are relevant in the context of shift work.

The sleep deprivation and psychological stress experienced by night-shift workers mirror the laboratory models used to evaluate lion's mane's efficacy.

Lion's mane addresses all three domains: it supports cognitive restoration, modulates inflammatory pathways, and rebalances neurotransmitter levels, all while improving subjective and objective sleep quality.

Moreover, the gut-brain axis may further amplify lion's mane's effects.

The bioavailability of its active compounds may be enhanced or modulated by intestinal microbiota.

While larger clinical trials remain necessary, early findings show strong and consistent results.

A clinical experiment showed that 8 weeks of oral lion's mane supplementation elevated circulating pro-BDNF and BDNF levels, correlating with improved mood and sleep scores.[338]

For shift workers battling anxiety, cognitive fog, or chronic sleep disturbances, lion's mane may offer a unique therapeutic tool, restoring not only sleep, but the cellular scaffolding required for resilience.

Lion's mane mushroom is more than a cognitive enhancer—it is a neurorestorative adaptogen. It doesn't push harder—it restores what exhaustion erodes. Not by forcing output, but by rebuilding capacity.

Blueprint Supplement Protocol: Lion's Mane Mushroom (Hericium erinaceus)

Category: Targeted Support (Neurotrophic Resilience, Cognitive Clarity, and Gut–Brain Modulation)

Form: Extracts derived from mycelium or fruiting body, ideally standardized to hericenones and erinacines, the bioactive compounds shown to support nerve growth factor and brain-derived neurotrophic factor.

- Clinical-grade options include Amyloban® 3399 and high-hericenone fruiting body extracts.

Dosing:

- 500–1,000 mg/day of a standardized extract for general neurocognitive support.

- Higher doses (up to 3,000 mg/day) may be used in therapeutic contexts for cognitive decline, neuropathy, or recovery from burnout.

Timing:

- Take in the morning or during early shift hours to enhance mood, focus, and circadian regulation without impairing sleep onset or overnight neural recovery.

Onset:

- Cognitive and mood benefits (clarity, processing speed, verbal fluency) may emerge within 2–4 weeks.

- Neurotrophic effects, including BDNF upregulation and synaptic plasticity, generally require 6–8 weeks of continuous use.

Pairing:

- Combine with magnesium, L-theanine, or PEA (palmitoylethanolamide) for stress recovery and parasympathetic support.

- Stack with probiotics (particularly *Bifidobacterium longum* or *Lactobacillus rhamnosus*) to enhance gut–brain communication and mood regulation.

Sleep, Mood, and the Shifted Brain

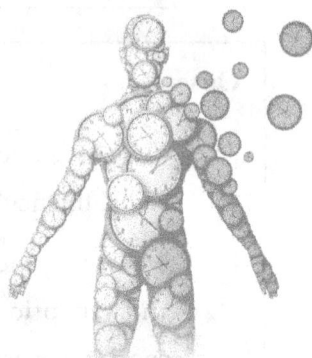

The fluorescent lights finally go dark. But the brain doesn't get the memo. The body is heavy. The world outside is silent. And still rest won't come. By the time they get home, the sun's already up. They've dodged death twice tonight, but now they're wired. The body is exhausted, but the thoughts are fast.

That's not insomnia.

That's circadian chaos.

This is the toll of a life lived out of rhythm.

For the night-shift nurse, the emergency responder, the factory worker watching the sun rise before rest has even begun, biology whispers what the schedule refuses to hear:

You are out of sync.

Sleep is more than the absence of wakefulness—it is an orchestrated process of repair, memory consolidation, emotional recalibration, and metabolic clearance.

When disrupted, as it often is in the lives of shift workers, the consequences cascade through the nervous system, immune network, and hormonal rhythms.

In this biologic tangle, astaxanthin, a carotenoid pigment derived from marine microalgae, has emerged as a potent candidate for intervention, targeting the shared molecular fault lines between sleep dysfunction and mood disorders.[339]

Astaxanthin (AST), a red-orange xanthophyll, crosses the blood-brain barrier and influences neurobiological pathways relevant to this disruption.[339] It suppresses oxidative stress by activating the Nrf2 antioxidant pathway, inhibits neuroinflammatory mediators like NF-κB and COX-2, and enhances BDNF expression, all of which are downregulated in individuals with MDD.[340]

Astaxanthin doesn't work overnight. In brain cells, it gradually reduces the expression of NMDA receptors, lowering excitotoxic stress that can wear neurons down shift after shift. Its strength is in steady protection—guarding mitochondrial energy and preserving brain resilience over time.[340] This NMDA blockade also modulates GABAergic interneurons and increases glutamate signaling through AMPA receptor insertion, further promoting synaptic resilience.[340]

The impact of AST on circadian biology is evident. In shift workers, misalignment isn't just felt—it's measurable. REM latency shortens. Sleep phases drift. Wakefulness arrives too soon. And mood, already frayed, follows that rhythm. AST increases Per2 expression and improves phase alignment. Though current evidence remains unpublished and preliminary, it suggests that AST may modulate circadian rhythm through its influence on BDNF, TrkB, and mTOR signaling pathways.[340]

Astrocytes, the brain's metabolic gatekeepers and circadian co-regulators, also respond to AST. It enhances astrocytic function by increasing TrkB-T1 expression and activating the ERK, Akt, and PKC pathway.[341] This protects astrocytes from apoptosis but also supports their role in modulating PER gene expression and calcium flux, core processes in circadian regulation.

These cellular effects begin to translate into human outcomes, though evidence is still early.

Clinical evidence, though limited, is promising. A small trial indicated that AST combined with zinc improved sleep onset latency.[342] Oral AST improved sleep patterns in patients with severe depression, but existing trials lack scale and rigor. Despite these gaps, AST's safety profile remains a major advantage. Approved as a nutraceutical, it integrates into functional foods and cosmetics and shows no evidence of toxicity.

Most studies use 4–12 mg daily, though optimal dosing for circadian health remains unestablished.

Astaxanthin is more than a potent antioxidant—it is an intelligent biological molecule capable of bridging the gap between sleep, mood, and circadian biology.

Despite its promise, orally ingested astaxanthin suffers from poor bioavailability—limited solubility, rapid metabolism, dependence on dietary fat, and even lifestyle factors like smoking all restrict how much ultimately reaches the bloodstream and, more importantly, the brain.[343]

However, advances in nanocarrier delivery systems, such as lipid-based or polymeric nanoparticles, may overcome these challenges.[343]

Its slow-release profile not only supports absorption, but may reinforce gut–brain signaling loops essential for circadian repair.[343] Enhancing its bioavailability without disrupting its slow release in the gut may preserve the microbiota interactions that contribute to its sleep and mood benefits.

For shift workers, who operate at the edge of chronodisruption, AST represents a promising, natural intervention. It addresses the silent inflammation, oxidative burden, and neurochemical drift that accompany a life lived against the biological clock.

In a world of chronic wakefulness, astaxanthin may be the small red molecule that restores not just sleep, but resilience.

Blueprint Supplement Protocol: Astaxanthin (AST)

Category: Targeted Support (Neuroinflammation, Sleep Quality, and Circadian Recovery)

Form: A potent xanthophyll carotenoid, typically derived from Haematococcus pluvialis microalgae and delivered in softgel capsules.

- Known for its lipophilic antioxidant properties and ability to cross the blood–brain and blood–retina barriers.

Dosing:

- 6–12 mg daily, with higher doses (10–12 mg) potentially offering greater benefit for neurocognitive resilience, inflammatory control, and sleep architecture.

Timing:

- Take with a fat-containing meal, ideally in the early evening or post-shift, to support sleep onset, circadian re-entrainment, and overnight recovery.

- Avoid dosing close to stimulants (e.g., caffeine) to maintain its phase-shifting potential.

Onset:

- Subjective improvements in sleep quality, visual clarity, and mood stability may begin within 2–4 weeks.

- Circadian and neurochemical effects (e.g., melatonin preservation, reduced oxidative load) accrue over long-term use.

Pairing:

- Combine with magnesium or zinc to support GABAergic tone, sleep latency, and hormonal recovery.

- May complement protocols involving omega-3s, vitamin D3, or PQQ for broader anti-inflammatory and mitochondrial synergy.

Clarity Before Sleep

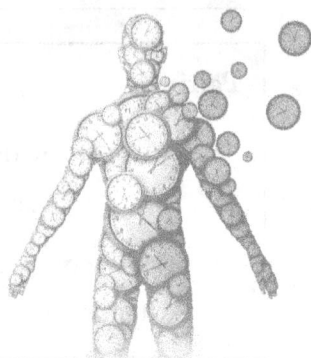

The clock reads 8:57 a.m. You've been off shift for an hour, but your brain is still pacing—wired, aching, awake. The bed welcomes you.

Sleep doesn't.

You stare at the ceiling, hoping your body will catch up to your exhaustion

Shift workers fight their biology each night, trying to sleep after schedules disrupt their internal clocks. It is not just the number of hours in bed that matter, but the ability to transition into rest, to quiet the mind and release the day.

In this context, palmitoylethanolamide (PEA) has emerged as a promising compound capable of improving sleep latency and next-day cognitive clarity without sedation or dependence.

PEA is an endogenous fatty acid amide produced by the body and believed to interact with the endocannabinoid system, modulating inflammation, pain, and neuronal signaling.[344]

Unlike traditional sleep medications that induce unconsciousness through blunt pharmacologic force—

PEA restores equilibrium.

It quiets inflammatory pathways.

Reduces hypersensitivity.

Promotes the conditions necessary for sleep to emerge, naturally.

In a randomized, double-blind, placebo-controlled trial, researchers assigned 103 adults with sleep disturbances to receive either 350 mg of Levagen+®, a bioavailable PEA formulation, or a placebo for eight weeks.

While both groups reported general improvements in sleep quality, likely due to increased sleep awareness, the PEA group experienced faster sleep onset, improved cognition upon waking, and reduced morning grogginess.[345]

PEA doesn't extend sleep.

It enhances the transition into it.

Researchers continue to explore the mechanisms behind these effects. PEA increases anandamide (AEA), an endocannabinoid that regulates calm and sleep.[346] It also influences mast cell activity, cytokine pathways, and pain perception.[347] Inflammation and hyperarousal are known disruptors of sleep, especially under chronic stress.

For shift workers, circadian disruption heightens inflammation and hyperarousal. PEA breaks this cycle by reducing both.

The study population included those with sleep disturbances but not primary insomnia, mirroring the shift work population. These individuals don't struggle to stay asleep—they struggle to fall asleep after night shifts or early morning transitions. Hypnotic drugs are not appropriate for them. PEA is.

Participants taking PEA felt more alert upon waking and demonstrated enhanced subjective cognition, a benefit as valuable as the sleep itself.[345]

PEA is approved as a nutraceutical and now enters functional foods, beverages, and cosmetics without evidence of toxicity. Its non-cannabinoid pathways, such as PPAR-α activation and NF-κB suppression, reduce both physical and neuroinflammatory resistance to rest.[345]

Most studies use 300–600 mg daily, often divided into one or two doses.

In a growing market of sleep aids, PEA represents a biologically compatible option—safe, flexible, and effective.

For those who don't lack tiredness but timing, it doesn't force sleep. It invites it. It doesn't cloud the mind.

It clears the way.

Clarity before sleep, and clarity when the next shift begins. Not sedation, but resilience—restored.

Blueprint Supplement Protocol:

Palmitoylethanolamide (PEA)

Category: Targeted Support (Sleep Initiation, Neuro-inflammation, and Post-Shift Recovery)

Form: An endogenous fatty acid amide, naturally produced in the body and available as an oral supplement.

- Look for enhanced-bioavailability formulations such as Levagen+®, which use dispersion technology to improve absorption and clinical efficacy.

Dosing:

- 350 mg once daily, taken 30–60 minutes before intended sleep.

- Effective for individuals with delayed sleep onset, circadian misalignment, or post-shift hyperarousal.

Timing:

- Ideal for use immediately after night shifts or during early-morning transitions when falling asleep is difficult.

- Can be used intermittently or in cycles during periods of disrupted sleep-wake schedules.

Onset:

- Sleep initiation and next-day cognitive clarity improvements are often noticed within 1–2 weeks.

- Additional anti-inflammatory and neuroprotective effects may accrue with ongoing use.

Pairing:

- Combine with blackout environments, magnesium glycinate, or L-theanine to deepen parasympathetic activation and promote sleep continuity.

- Avoid combining with sedative-hypnotic medications (e.g., benzodiazepines, Z-drugs) without clinical supervision.

Resetting The
Clock From Within

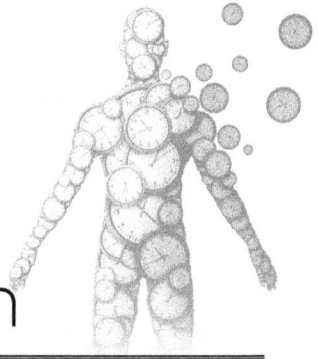

By the end of a third consecutive night shift, the body was wide awake, while the brain begged for rest. Stepping into the morning light, the outcome was predictable: a two-hour battle to fall asleep, five restless hours in bed, and a fog that wouldn't lift before the next night on the floor. Light remains the most potent cue for circadian entrainment, and as discussed earlier, tools like bright-light exposure or dawn simulation lamps help reset the clock. But what if you could enhance that signal from the inside out?

A small molecule, L-serine, might help the body interpret morning light not as a cue to stay awake, but as a signal to reset.

Shift work disconnects the body from its environment, dismantling internal synchrony. The body's internal clock, governed by the suprachiasmatic nuclei of the hypothalamus, requires external cues, particularly light, to maintain alignment with the 24-hour day. When this coordination falters, sleep-wake cycles fragment, alertness wanes, and disease risk rises.[348]

L-serine, a non-essential amino acid classified as Generally Recognized as Safe by the FDA, has shown the potential to enhance light-induced phase resetting of the circadian clock.[348] In both mice and humans, ingestion of L-serine prior to light exposure resulted in measurable advances in circadian phase, as evidenced by accelerated shifts in locomotor activity in mice and earlier dim-light melatonin onset (DLMO) in humans.[349]

L-serine does not function as a primary synchronizer. Its effect on the circadian system emerges when paired with light, where it amplifies light's impact rather than initiating alignment on its own.

In animal studies, timing and delivery mattered: concentrated doses before rest worked, while scattered intake diluted the effect. These findings suggest that L-serine might influence brain pathways that use GABA, not just in the SCN (the body's master clock), but also in other areas like the intergeniculate leaflet and raphe nuclei, regions that help regulate how light affects the body's internal clock.[349]

L-serine also alters long-term expression patterns of clock genes. This delayed action supports its role in facilitating re-entrainment following abrupt shifts in the light-dark cycle. In mice subjected to a simulated jet lag (a 6-hour light advance), L-serine ingestion before the shift significantly reduced the time required to realign circadian activity rhythms.[350]

These results translate to human physiology. In a double-blind crossover study, participants who consumed 3 grams of L-serine before bedtime experienced a greater phase advance of DLMO following bright light exposure the next morning, compared to placebo.[350] The observed advance (~26 minutes) was double that of the placebo group and fell well within the expected range based on established phase response curves for morning light.

Most studies use around 3 grams nightly, timed just before bed, though shift-specific protocols are still emerging.

L-serine had no adverse effects on sleep quality or daytime alertness and showed a trend toward improved psychomotor vigilance task (PVT) scores, suggesting potential benefits for next-day performance.[351]

The effectiveness of L-serine hinges on timing and delivery. In murine studies, gavage (forced oral administration) produced consistent effects, whereas delivery via drinking water did not. The distinction appears to lie in pharmacokinetics: consistent low-dose exposure may desensitize or distribute L-serine's impact across the light cycle, diminishing its ability to prime a specific phase response.[350] In contrast, timed ingestion just before bedtime concentrates its action around the critical early morning phase advance window.

L-serine influences circadian biology through its interaction with astrocytes, cells that regulate the molecular clock.[350] Astrocyte dysfunction marks major depressive disorder and links directly to sleep disruption and altered glutamate signaling.[352] L-serine supports astrocyte metabolism and may influence clock gene expression via BDNF-TrkB-Akt and mTOR pathways.[351]

These pathways also regulate neuroplasticity, linking L-serine's chronobiologic effects to potential mood and cognition benefits, especially when combined with light exposure. These same astrocytic pathways, disrupted in mood disorders, suggest L-serine may hold dual benefits: for rhythm and for emotional resilience.

Taken together, the evidence positions L-serine as a functional chrononutrient: a non-pharmacologic agent that, when paired with appropriately timed light exposure, can accelerate circadian realignment, support alertness, and prevent downstream effects of circadian misalignment such as mood disorders and metabolic dysfunction.

For shift workers who struggle not only to sleep but to synchronize, L-serine offers something rare: a biological nudge, not to sleep longer, but to sleep smarter. Not to override the clock, but to reintroduce rhythm. For shift workers, L-serine isn't a sedative—it's a synchronizer. A way to reclaim rhythm when the world pulls you off time.

Blueprint Supplement Protocol: L-serine

Category: Targeted Support (Circadian Phase Shifting and Sleep-Wake Realignment)

Form: A non-essential amino acid, available in powder or capsule form.

- Often used in chronobiology protocols to support circadian re-entrainment in shift workers or those experiencing jet lag.

Dosing:

- 3 grams once daily, taken consistently to support phase-shifted sleep onset and circadian adaptation.

Timing:

- Ingest 30–60 minutes before intended bedtime, ideally prior to next-morning light exposure.

- Best suited for use on transition days or during circadian misalignment, particularly when advancing the sleep phase is required.

Onset:

- Circadian effects typically begin after several days of use when paired with bright morning light (>5,000 lux).

- Measurable phase advances in melatonin onset and sleep timing are often observed within one week.

Pairing:

- Must be paired with bright morning light to be effective— not recommended as a standalone intervention.

- May also be used in combination with magnesium or apigenin to improve sleep architecture during circadian transitions.

Subtle stimulation behind the Scenes

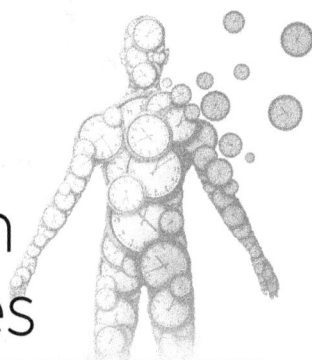

It's 4:00 a.m. in the dim glow of a hospital breakroom. A night-shift nurse unwraps a square of dark chocolate, not for hunger, but for hope. Caffeine is off-limits this late in the shift.

The chocolate is a gamble. Not a solution, just something to hold the line.

In the pharmacological toolkit of the shift worker, caffeine often takes center stage—fast, predictable, and widely understood.

But beneath the surface of caffeinated choices lies a quieter compound: theobromine.

Theobromine, a methylxanthine present in chocolate and similar foods, enters the diet without conscious choice. Where caffeine acts like a spotlight—sharp, immediate, directional—theobromine is background noise. Constant. Mild. Unnoticed, until it accumulates. Like slowly filling a cup under a dripping tap until it spills.

Its effects, while milder than caffeine, are dose-dependent— sometimes beneficial, sometimes disruptive.

At lower intakes (around 250 mg), effects are subtle. At higher doses, above 500 mg, performance begins to degrade, and by 1000 mg, alertness declines instead of sharpens.[353]

The structure mimics caffeine. The stimulation does not. If your nighttime routine includes dark chocolate, energy bars, or cocoa protein powders, total theobromine intake may exceed 400–600 mg without conscious intention.

In shift workers already navigating misalignment and sleep debt, that distinction matters.

Unlike caffeine, which sharpens alertness, high-dose theobromine dulls it, slowing reaction time, increasing heart rate, and raising discomfort.[354]

Mood effects follow a similar curve. Mild doses feel neutral or faintly pleasant; high doses can tip into irritability, anxiety, even dislike.

And while caffeine lowers blood pressure, theobromine raises heart rate without affecting pressure—a subtle physiological ripple, but one worth noting for those with cardiovascular strain.[353]

Genetics complicate the picture: variations in the ADORA2A gene alter sensitivity, meaning one worker's calm may be another's anxiety.[355]

Chocolate cravings? Often blamed on theobromine. But the real driver may be the sugar-fat-caffeine combo, not this compound alone.[356]

Theobromine is not a stimulant. It's a whisper, not a jolt. In a life built on artificial wakefulness, that whisper can blur the line between help and harm.

For shift workers, it's not about cutting chocolate, but about understanding the context.

Theobromine won't crash cognition like overused caffeine. But it won't lift it, either, not beyond a point.

Its role? Minor. Peripheral. But worth knowing.

Because in the fog of fatigue, not every compound clears the air.

Some only thicken it—and knowing the difference can mean the line between a coping ritual and a hidden liability.

Blueprint Supplement Protocol: Theobromine

Category: Targeted Support (Mild Stimulant Modulation and Early-Shift Alertness)

Form: A naturally occurring methylxanthine found in cocoa, dark chocolate, and select teas; also available as capsule or powdered extract.

- Compared to caffeine, theobromine has a gentler onset, longer half-life, and less pronounced central stimulation.

Dosing:

- 100–250 mg produces subtle stimulant and vasodilatory effects.

- Doses exceeding 500 mg may impair mood, focus, or sleep quality, particularly in stimulant-sensitive individuals.

Timing:

- Best used during the first third of a shift to promote early alertness without interfering with downstream sleep onset.

- Avoid dosing during the final third of a shift, especially when transitioning to post-shift recovery sleep.

Onset:

- Subtle effects (e.g., wakefulness, vascular tone, respiratory drive) typically begin within 30–60 minutes.

- Peak alerting impact occurs within 1–2 hours, depending on dose, food intake, and individual metabolism.

Pairing:

- May be cautiously paired with caffeine early in the shift for balanced alertness.

- Avoid combining with other stimulants late in the shift block to prevent sleep fragmentation or circadian delay.

PART III

Precision
That Requires
Partnership

Some tools work deeper, modulating neurotransmitters, hormones, or cellular energy systems in ways that can be powerful, but not always predictable.

This section explores those compounds. Ones that may offer meaningful benefit in buffering against extreme fatigue, cognitive burnout, or long-term physiological strain, but carry a greater potential for interaction, side effects, or misapplication. These aren't supplements to casually layer on.

They're advanced interventions, best approached with context, timing, and clinical guidance.

And just like everything in this book: you are not obligated to take them. There is no badge for trying everything. In fact, the wiser path is often restraint. If something here piques your interest, bring it to your provider. Use this chapter as a conversation starter, not a prescription.

Even if you never touch them, understanding how they work deepens your knowledge of your own biology.

Because when the terrain gets more complex, the tools must get more precise. And precision, at this level, requires partnership, not improvisation.

A Pharmacologic
Nudge

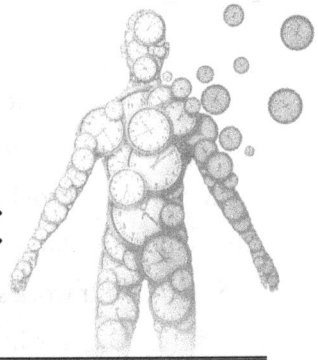

It's 2:47 a.m. on night three of four. A paramedic leans forward, eyes dry, hands steady, brain lagging behind the siren. Alertness isn't optional. But tonight, it won't arrive on its own.

Shift workers don't just battle fatigue—they battle physiology. And when non-pharmacologic tools like nutrition, light, and sleep hygiene aren't enough, the question becomes: What then?

This section turns to chemistry, not as a first resort, but as a form of reinforcement. And at the pharmacologic tier, few tools have received as much clinical attention for shift work as modafinil, a prescription-only wakefulness agent that doesn't override the clock, but supports those living against it.

Here, we explore medications that support alertness, rest, mood stability, and rhythm restoration in those living out of sync. These are not cures. They are bridges—used wisely, they can reconnect the body to a rhythm it has lost.

In the misaligned physiology of shift work, where the circadian clock remains fixed while the world demands flexibility, alertness at night can become a biological impossibility. When foundational strategies like light exposure, structured sleep, and recovery routines fail to realign circadian rhythm, pharmacologic tools such as modafinil enter the equation, not to cure misalignment, but to push the brain toward wakefulness during biologically low-alert states.

Modafinil (Provigil) is a wake-promoting agent approved for narcolepsy and later extended for use in obstructive sleep apnea (OSA) and shift work sleep disorder.[357] Unlike traditional stimulants, modafinil does not induce hyperarousal.[357] Its mechanism remains unclear, but it raises extracellular dopamine and norepinephrine levels and activates histamine and orexin pathways in the hypothalamus.[357]

The result is enhanced alertness without classic stimulant side effects like jitteriness or significant rebound fatigue. Modafinil's unique pharmacologic profile sharpens attention without overstimulating the brain, making it especially effective for shift workers.

Modafinil is typically prescribed at 200 mg once daily, though doses up to 400 mg are sometimes used under supervision.[357]

In a landmark randomized controlled trial involving over two hundred night-shift workers diagnosed with SWSD, 200 mg of modafinil taken at the start of the night shift led to significant statistical, but modest clinical, improvements.[358] Participants experienced increased nighttime sleep latency (an indicator of reduced sleepiness), fewer lapses of attention during psychomotor vigilance testing, and improved cognitive function upon waking.[358]

Notably, modafinil reduced the number of reported accidents and near misses during the morning commute, a finding with real-world safety implications.[359]

However, these benefits were bounded. Treated participants remained excessively sleepy, with mean sleep latencies well below normal alertness thresholds. Even on modafinil, participants were alert enough to function, but still at risk in safety-critical settings.

Unlike light or melatonin, modafinil does not shift the circadian clock, it only masks its resistance to wakefulness. In this way, modafinil is not a tool of correction, but of mitigation.

Tolerability is favorable. The most reported side effect is headache, and modafinil does not appear to impair post-shift daytime sleep, making it a viable option for individuals who require both nocturnal alertness and daytime recovery.[358] However, long-term data in shift work populations remain limited. The trial durations were short, typically three months, and do not capture the effects of chronic use in rotating or variable shift schedules.

Despite these limitations, modafinil has become a cornerstone pharmacologic intervention in SWSD.[360] It is relevant for those who cannot avoid overnight schedules but are biologically incapable of maintaining performance across them. And yet, its use underscores a deeper truth: pharmacology can supplement, but not replace, circadian alignment. Medications like modafinil work best when paired with strategic naps, light exposure, and carefully protected sleep windows. Without these, they are merely patches on a leaking system.

As shift work becomes the norm rather than the exception, pharmacologic scaffolding, like modafinil, will play a growing role. It offers relief, not resolution. A chemical boost for biological misalignment. But no pill can replace sleep. No stimulant rewires the clock.

Used wisely, it's a scaffold. Not a cure, not a substitute for rhythm, but a partner in holding the line when biology resists.

Blueprint Supplement Protocol: Modafinil (Provigil®)

Category: Precision Support (Wakefulness Promotion and Shift Performance)

Form: A prescription-only eugeroic (wakefulness-promoting agent), available in 100 mg and 200 mg tablets.

- Approved for conditions such as shift work sleep disorder, narcolepsy, and obstructive sleep apnea-related hypersomnia.

Dosing:

- Standard clinical dose: 200 mg once daily, taken 30–60 minutes before the start of a night shift.

- May be adjusted under medical supervision based on tolerance, duration of shifts, or coexisting conditions.

Timing:

- Administer just before shift start to sustain wakefulness during biologically low-alert hours (typically 11 p.m. to 6 a.m.).

- Avoid use too late in the shift to prevent residual stimulation and delayed sleep onset post-shift.

Onset:

- Alertness effects generally begin within 1–2 hours of ingestion.

- Duration of action is 12–15 hours, making precise timing essential to avoid interference with recovery sleep.

Pairing:

- For best outcomes, pair with:
  - Bright light exposure at shift onset.
  - Prophylactic napping before night shifts.
  - Aggressive sleep protection post-shift (e.g., blackout curtains, sleep masks, melatonin if appropriate).

- Does not replace circadian alignment strategies and may not be appropriate for long-term or daily use without careful oversight.

Strategies Without Stimulants

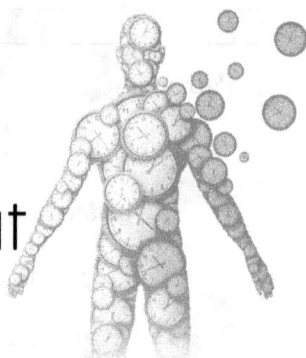

It's 5:00 a.m. Their eyes are open, but they're not fully awake. Their limbs are heavy, their mind clouded with dream fragments—and they still have two hours left on shift. What's happening isn't just fatigue. It's intrusion.

In the landscape of pharmacologic wakefulness, most agents rely on brute force—stimulating dopamine release, overriding fatigue, or temporarily blunting the brain's push toward sleep.

Pitolisant (Wakix) offers something different. It does not sedate or stimulate—it recalibrates. As a selective histamine H3 receptor antagonist, it works upstream of other neurotransmitters, increasing histamine release while indirectly enhancing other wake-promoting systems.[361]

Approved for the treatment of excessive daytime sleepiness (EDS) and cataplexy in narcolepsy, pitolisant introduces a unique mechanism to a space long dominated by dopaminergic stimulants and offers a potential model for therapies addressing shift work–related sleepiness.[362]

By blocking presynaptic H3 autoreceptors, pitolisant increases the release of histamine in the brain, a neurotransmitter intricately linked to sleep-wake regulation.[370]

What makes pitolisant distinct is its capacity to promote wakefulness without triggering the reward system. Unlike amphetamines or modafinil, it does not elevate dopamine in the nucleus accumbens, a brain region associated with addiction and reinforcement. In clinical studies, pitolisant demonstrated minimal to no abuse potential, and it remains unscheduled by the DEA, a rarity among wake-promoting compounds.[369,370]

In pooled clinical trials, pitolisant significantly improved both subjective and objective measures of alertness.

"I don't feel wired—I feel steady. Like I have my brain back without the crash."— Night-shift pharmacist

Epworth Sleepiness Scale (ESS) scores declined, and Maintenance of Wakefulness Test (MWT) results improved, often within the 2–3 week titration phase.[363] Pitolisant is typically initiated at 8.9 mg daily and titrated up to 35.6 mg based on response and tolerability. Patients with high symptom burden—ESS ≥16, sleep latency <8 minutes, or frequent cataplexy—saw outcomes comparable to traditional agents, but without stimulant trade-offs.

Yet response isn't uniform. Some individuals improve quickly, others need time. Pitolisant works slowly and subtly—not as a jolt, but a recalibration.

Pitolisant does not function by force. It modulates. It nudges the brain's internal wake-promoting systems, enhancing regulatory networks rather than overriding them. This may explain its impact on REM intrusions and its stabilizing effects on cataplexy.

Despite its novelty and promise, pitolisant is not a universal solution. It works best as part of a comprehensive treatment approach, one that includes behavioral optimization, sleep hygiene, structured napping, and, where necessary, treatment of coexisting disorders like sleep apnea. The future of narcolepsy treatment may lie not in the blunt suppression of symptoms, but in precision modulation of sleep-wake networks, and pitolisant represents a meaningful step in that direction.

Pitolisant is non-sedating, non-stimulating, and non-reinforcing, a rare trifecta in the pharmacologic management of narcolepsy. For patients living in the gray zone between wake and sleep, where alertness fades and muscle tone collapses without warning, pitolisant offers a way to stabilize the instability, not perfectly, but meaningfully.

And for those living out of sync, pitolisant offers not just wakefulness, but the restoration of subtle clarity—the kind that steadies rather than stimulates. The kind that doesn't shout. It listens. And sometimes, that listening can mean survival.

Blueprint Supplement Protocol: Pitolisant (Wakix®)

Category: Precision Support (Histaminergic Activation and Excessive Sleepiness Reduction)

Form: A prescription H3 receptor inverse agonist, available in 4.5 mg and 18 mg tablets.

- Approved for the treatment of excessive daytime sleepiness and cataplexy in narcolepsy, with growing off-label interest for shift work sleep disorder.

Dosing:

- Initiate at 8.9 mg once daily.
- Titrate weekly based on clinical response and tolerability, up to a maximum dose of 35.6 mg/day.
- Requires gradual up-titration to minimize side effects and optimize CNS adaptation.

Timing:

- Take in the morning to align with natural wake cycles and minimize risk of delayed sleep onset or insomnia.
- Not recommended for mid- or late-shift dosing due to long half-life (~10–12 hours).

Onset:

- Clinical improvements in wakefulness, particularly in EDS, are often observed within 2–3 weeks.
- Full therapeutic effects may take several weeks, especially when titrated conservatively.

Pairing:

- Best used as part of a comprehensive strategy including:

  – Behavioral interventions (light exposure, sleep hygiene, cognitive pacing).

  – Management of underlying sleep disorders (e.g., OSA, circadian rhythm disorders).

  – Routine provider monitoring to assess titration response and safety markers.

PART IV

Where the
Tradeoffs Live

Performance Without Alignment

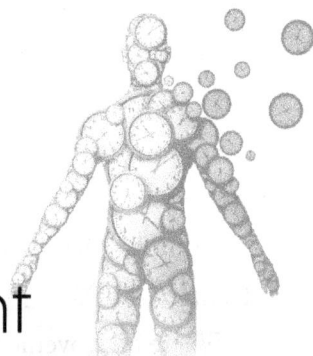

Just before dawn, a trauma nurse walks to their car after a 12-hour night shift. The highway is empty. The body—heavy. The brain—fogged. They've driven this route a hundred times.

Halfway home, their eyes close for two seconds—just two. When they open, they've drifted into the shoulder.

This isn't about fatigue anymore. It's about safety.

In the twilight hours of the biological night, when the body insists on sleep, but the job demands alertness, the consequences of cognitive failure are high. The need for pharmacologic support becomes less about enhancing productivity and more about preserving function—and sometimes, safety.

To protect workers during these dangerous inflection points, pharmacologic scaffolding like armodafinil has emerged, not as a stimulant, but as a buffer. Armodafinil (Nuvigil®) is a wake-promoting agent structurally related to modafinil, but pharmacologically refined. It contains only the R-enantiomer of modafinil, the longer-lasting isomer, which provides more sustained plasma levels and greater coverage during the later stages of the night shift and the early morning commute, when sleep pressure is most intense.[364] In controlled studies, 150 mg of armodafinil administered before a night shift improved mean sleep latency, reduced subjective sleepiness, and enhanced attention and memory without impairing daytime sleep or vital signs.[365]

Armodafinil is typically prescribed at 150–250 mg before the start of a night shift.

These improvements were not abstract—they translated to fewer unintended sleep episodes, fewer mistakes at work, and a trend toward reduced near-miss accidents while commuting.[361] Importantly, armodafinil increased mean sleep latency beyond the threshold that defines severe sleepiness, though patients remained impaired.[361]

Cognitive testing revealed that armodafinil improved sustained attention, episodic memory, and reaction time.[360]

"I can't trust my reflexes after 4 a.m. anymore—armodafinil is the only thing keeping me from falling asleep on the drive."

— ER nurse, night shift

Unlike caffeine, which stimulates broadly and temporarily, armodafinil seemed to enhance accuracy as well as speed, suggesting improvements not just in speed, but in accuracy of alert processing.[361] These modest gains carried clinical relevance. Clinicians use comparable reductions in sleep latency to justify wake-promoting medications in disorders like narcolepsy and obstructive sleep apnea, where maintaining alertness forms the cornerstone of treatment.

Like modafinil, armodafinil does not realign the circadian clock—it overrides sleep pressure without correcting misalignment.

Its benefit is one of performance preservation during circadian misalignment, not correction of the misalignment itself. This compound does not cure SWSD. It functions as a chemical scaffold, supporting wakefulness during key hours while leaving the underlying circadian disruption untouched.

Armodafinil produces minimal adverse effects in most users. The most common side effects include headache and nausea.[361] It does not impair daytime recovery sleep and has not been associated with significant changes in ECG, laboratory values, or vital signs in most studies. Elevated blood pressure and heart rate appear inconsistently and require close monitoring in individuals with cardiovascular risk.[361]

Armodafinil delivers measurable benefits for many, but not all, shift workers. A subset of patients remained sleepy even after treatment, reinforcing the idea that pharmacologic wakefulness should be one component of a broader strategy. That strategy must include screening for comorbid sleep disorders (e.g., OSA, narcolepsy), structured light exposure, scheduled recovery periods, workplace fatigue protocols, and education on sleep hygiene and circadian principles. No pill can restore alignment in a life lived out of rhythm.

In industries like healthcare, transportation, and emergency services, where errors carry high stakes, armodafinil may reduce risk. But it should never replace structural protections like appropriate scheduling, protected breaks, or circadian-informed shift design. Where organizational policy falls short, armodafinil can function as a compensatory tool. But it cannot compensate for a system built to ignore biology.

Pharmacology can help, sometimes profoundly. But for the shift worker, alignment remains the true antidote. Armodafinil may sharpen performance. It may delay failure. But rhythm, protected and reclaimed, is what sustains survival.

THE SHIFT WORKERS PARADOX

Blueprint Supplement Protocol:
Armodafinil (Nuvigil®)

Category: Precision Support (Extended Wakefulness and Shift Optimization)

Form: A prescription eugeroic, available as 150 mg tablets.

- The R-enantiomer of modafinil, armodafinil provides a longer duration of effect with a more gradual offset, making it well-suited for extended shift coverage.

Dosing:

- Standard dose: 150 mg once daily, taken 30–60 minutes prior to the start of a night shift.

- Dosage adjustments should be made under clinical supervision, particularly for those with renal impairment or coexisting conditions.

Timing:

- Administer just before shift onset to sustain wakefulness through the core of the circadian nadir (typically 2–6 a.m.).

- May provide more even coverage than modafinil in longer or more demanding shifts.

Onset:

- Subjective alertness improvements typically begin within 1–2 hours.

- Peak plasma levels are achieved around 2 hours post-dose, with a duration of action that may extend beyond 14 hours.

Pairing:

- For optimal impact:

  - Combine with strategic light exposure (5,000–10,000 lux) early in the shift.

  - Ensure protected post-shift recovery sleep with blackout environments and, if needed, circadian-phase tools like melatonin.

  - Screen for and manage coexisting sleep disorders such as obstructive sleep apnea or narcolepsy, which may alter response and risk profile.

Wakefulness
When Nature Fails

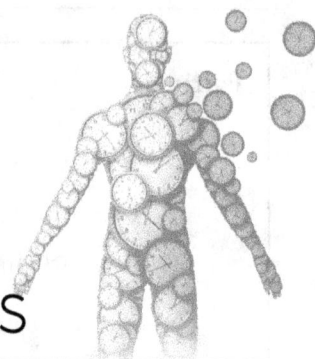

There comes a point in shift work when the system breaks. When sleep hygiene tips, blue light filters, and scheduled naps feel like whispers against a freight train. Shift workers don't just fight fatigue, they endure biological sabotage. The brain pleads for sleep. The clock demands performance.

And the body is caught in between—overruled, overstretched, and out of rhythm.

In these moments, what's needed is not another lecture about routine, but a pharmacologic lifeline. Not to fix the misalignment, because some rhythms can't be rescued in real time, but to hold the line. Solriamfetol is that line. A potential pharmaceutical scaffold designed not for stimulation, but for survival, when alertness can no longer be willed into existence.

Shift work demands what the human body never evolved to do: stay alert through darkness, sleep through daylight, and perform under fatigue. Behavioral and circadian strategies help, but beyond a certain threshold, physiology stops responding to coaching. In these cases, pharmacologic scaffolding holds the system upright—not to repair the clock, but to stabilize function when realignment remains out of reach.

Solriamfetol is one of the newest tools in this category. A dual dopamine and norepinephrine reuptake inhibitor, solriamfetol is also a TAAR1 agonist, a novel mechanism designed not to sedate or stimulate in the traditional sense, but to support wakefulness with precision.[366] Already approved for the treatment of excessive daytime sleepiness in obstructive sleep apnea and narcolepsy, solriamfetol is now under investigation for a new frontier: excessive sleepiness associated with shift work sleep disorder.[363] The FDA offered early guidance, and a Phase 3 trial now moves forward under clear regulatory direction.

The need is substantial. One third of Americans perform shift work, and up to 43% may meet clinical criteria for SWSD.[367] These individuals report high rates of insomnia, daytime impairment, and excessive nighttime sleepiness. At its worst, this sleepiness is not subtle—it includes falling asleep on the job or behind the wheel, with serious public health consequences.

As we covered in previous chapters, available pharmacologic options include modafinil and armodafinil, both wakefulness-promoting agents approved for the treatment of shift work sleep disorder. While they can improve alertness and reduce sleepiness during night shifts, their effects are symptomatic, not curative.

Though effective, these agents may not sustain alertness through the entire shift. Their effects can fade in the final hours, precisely when cognitive performance is most vulnerable. Solriamfetol helps fill that gap, offering a longer and more stable half-life for extended coverage across the shift span.

Clinical data from OSA populations, who often share the same EDS profile as shift workers, have been encouraging. That promise isn't theoretical—it's been tested. In a Phase 3 study, solriamfetol significantly increased wakefulness (as measured by the Maintenance of Wakefulness Test) and reduced subjective sleepiness (Epworth Sleepiness Scale).[368] Improvements extended beyond symptoms: patients also experienced enhanced quality of life, daily functioning, and work productivity, particularly at the 150 mg dose.[365] These gains included better role function, reduced presenteeism, and fewer impairments in social and physical activity.[365,366]

"I don't want to rely on meds, but when I'm rounding at 6 a.m. and my brain wants to sleep, solriamfetol keeps me sharp enough to keep patients safe." — Critical care nurse, rotating nights

What sets solriamfetol apart is not just its efficacy, but its practical versatility. Unlike traditional stimulants such as amphetamines or methylphenidate, which carry high abuse potential and can trigger rebound hypersomnia, solriamfetol's mechanism allows for targeted wakefulness with lower risk.

Compared to modafinil, it demonstrates more sustained plasma levels and may offer improved performance in the late hours of extended wakefulness, a common vulnerability in SWSD.[369]

Solriamfetol meets a critical standard: tolerability. Across clinical trials, the most commonly reported side effects were headache and nausea, with no serious cardiovascular events observed.[370] More importantly, solriamfetol preserved scheduled daytime sleep, an essential requirement for any agent used in the context of circadian misalignment.

However, studies did document modest increases in heart rate and blood pressure, highlighting the importance of appropriate monitoring.[367]

It is important to note that solriamfetol, like all pharmacologic interventions, does not realign circadian rhythms. It does not advance melatonin onset or synchronize sleep-wake timing. Its role is compensatory: to reduce sleep propensity when the body insists on shutting down. Use it within a broader therapeutic framework that includes circadian education, targeted light exposure, structured naps, and clinical screening for conditions such as obstructive sleep apnea, narcolepsy, or restless legs syndrome.

Looking forward, solriamfetol offers promising potential for shift workers. If approved, it would become only the third agent recognized for SWSD, a condition underdiagnosed despite its high burden of morbidity, performance impairment, and public risk.[371] Its use could support industries where fatigue-related errors carry high consequences: healthcare, transportation, emergency response.

Solriamfetol does not erase the toll of misaligned biology, but it can buy clarity when the body shuts down. For those forced to operate beyond nature's boundaries, it offers something rare: sustainable wakefulness in a system still asking for sleep.

Solriamfetol won't retune the rhythm. But it lets you keep playing—until the body catches up.

Blueprint Supplement Protocol:
Solriamfetol (Sunosi®)

Category: Precision Support (Wakefulness Maintenance and Dopaminergic/Noradrenergic Activation)

Form: A prescription dual-acting dopamine/norepinephrine reuptake inhibitor (DNRI), available in 75 mg and 150 mg tablets.

- Approved for excessive daytime sleepiness associated with shift work sleep disorder, obstructive sleep apnea, and narcolepsy.

Dosing:

- Start with 75 mg once daily, taken shortly after waking.

- Dose may be increased to 150 mg/day based on clinical response and tolerability.

- Higher doses are not typically associated with improved effect and may increase side-effect risk.

Timing:

- Administer soon after waking (day or night) to align with biological alerting windows and prevent interference with subsequent sleep cycles.

- Not intended for use in the middle or end of a shift due to its long half-life (~7 hours).

Onset:

- Subjective improvements in alertness often appear within the first few days.

- Full therapeutic effect may take 1–2 weeks of consistent use.

Pairing:

- Use in conjunction with:

  - Evidence-based sleep hygiene protocols.

  - Circadian rhythm education and timing awareness.

  - Clinical screening for underlying sleep disorders (e.g., OSA, narcolepsy, insomnia), which may alter efficacy and risk profile.

Pharmacological Tension

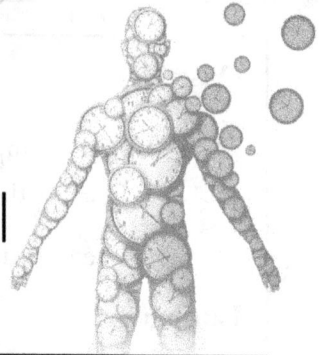

It's 4:30 a.m. The ED is quiet for now. A nurse pops a half-tab of methylphenidate, not to get ahead, but to make it home without crashing. They've used it all week, but today, the sleep won't come.

Stimulants offer a seductive promise: enhanced alertness, sharpened focus, and sustained performance. For shift workers, these aren't luxuries—they're survival tools. Among them, methylphenidate (MPH) remains one of the most studied—and most polarizing.

But they come with a physiological, and sometimes psychological, cost.

Few consequences of shift work rival the damage of chronic sleep loss.

Stimulant medications like MPH expose this conflict. They sharpen focus. They suppress fatigue.

But they do so by interfering with the brain's natural descent into sleep. The question isn't if they impair sleep, but when, how much, and in whom.

Studies evaluating stimulant effects on sleep reveal a landscape of inconsistency. Trials show that late-afternoon or evening dosing delays sleep onset.[372,373] Others find no significant difference between midday and 4 p.m. administration. Flexible dosing protocols, often titrated to effect, complicate these findings.

In real-world use, dosing often halts when sleep disturbances appear or when perceived benefits plateau, obscuring clearer dose-response patterns in research.

Sleep response also shifts over time. Early in use, stimulant-related insomnia may appear pronounced, only to improve as tolerance builds or dosing stabilizes. Yet this adaptation does not always signal resolution. Rebound insomnia, the abrupt return of fatigue or wakefulness when the drug wears off, can make it paradoxically harder to fall asleep after a full night of pharmacologically sustained alertness.[374]

Anecdotal reports from shift workers further complicate this picture. Stimulant users describe improved sleep following low-dose stimulant use when that use helps reduce anxious rumination or excessive mental noise.[375] In others, the ability to remain focused during night shifts comes at the expense of delayed sleep onset, fragmented rest, or shallow early morning sleep.

"I can focus through the chaos, but I know I'm trading that for four hours of staring at the ceiling when I get home."— Night-shift physician

Objective sleep measures underscore this variability. In one study, stimulant use delayed sleep onset by 20 to 30 minutes compared to placebo.[373] But these averages mask wide inter-individual variability.

Some shift workers tolerate stimulants without sleep disruption. For others, even modest doses destabilize rest. Extended-release formulations and split-dose strategies, sometimes necessary for long shifts, introduce further complexity, as sleep disruption does not always follow predictable patterns based on dose or timing alone.

Shift workers face a unique vulnerability. Their circadian system is already misaligned. Adding pharmacologic alertness may further widen the gap between biological need and external demand.

For those who rely on stimulants during night shifts or rotating schedules, this misalignment deepens. Sleep onset becomes more difficult, and the quality of rest suffers. Over time, even mild disruptions accumulate, reducing the brain's ability to recover and compounding fatigue across shift cycles.

Before starting stimulant therapy, it is essential to assess sleep health. Shift workers frequently experience undiagnosed circadian rhythm disorders, insufficient sleep, or environmental barriers to rest. Clinicians should rule out primary sleep disorders—such as obstructive sleep apnea, restless legs syndrome, or delayed sleep phase—that may compound stimulant-related insomnia. Baseline measurements of sleep duration, variability, and onset can help distinguish medication effects from underlying dysfunction.

Evening stimulant use, though sometimes necessary, requires caution. The benefits of wakefulness come with a tradeoff: delayed recovery, reduced sleep depth, and next-day fatigue. For shift workers, sleep is not a luxury or secondary concern. It is the foundation of safety, resilience, and long-term health. A stimulant regimen that enhances alertness but undermines sleep may offer short-term gains while accelerating long-term decline.

Individual response remains variable. There are individuals who tolerate stimulants well and recover. Others report persistent insomnia, mood disruption, or early morning exhaustion.[373] Predictors of sensitivity include prior sleep difficulties, younger age, higher doses, and dosing late in the waking period.[373] But exceptions abound—

workers who perform best with split dosing, or those whose sleep improves with low-dose pharmacologic support.

Until personalized protocols emerge, the clinical approach must prioritize vigilance. Stimulants are not benign. For some, they deliver clarity and control. For others, they disrupt rest and derail recovery. In shift work, where sleep is already scarce and fragile, this distinction becomes critical.

In shift work, where sleep is already scarce and fragile, this tension becomes the pivot point between performance and collapse. And the decision to medicate must begin with sleep, not end with it. In the end, performance depends on sleep. Survival depends on it.

The consequences of circadian disruption don't end with sleep. They extend deeper, into immunity itself.

Vaccine Response in Shift Workers

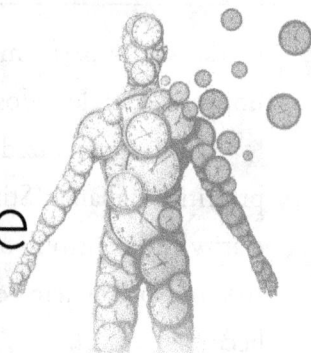

It was 3 a.m. in the emergency department when a veteran night-shift nurse mentioned, almost offhandedly, that she'd just finished her third hepatitis B vaccination. She had followed every protocol. Never missed a dose. No chronic illness, no known risk factors.

And yet she still hadn't seroconverted. Her antibody test came back negative. Again.

The medicine had done its job. Her biology hadn't.

What she did have was a decade of rotating night shifts, broken sleep, and vitamin D levels flagged as deficient in lab after lab.

Not an error. A pattern.

A pattern that points to a deeper biological vulnerability, one invisible on the clock-in sheet but written all over the immune system.

This is the quiet cost of shift work—not just fatigue, but a compromised ability to respond. Even to protection. What happened to her wasn't an anomaly, it was a biologically predictable outcome.

In the clinical landscape of immunization, a vaccine is only as effective as the body's ability to respond to it. In most people, standard vaccinations trigger the immune system to form antibodies, establish memory, and reduce the risk of future illness. But for shift workers, the biology behind this expectation does not always hold. Disrupted circadian rhythms, chronic sleep deprivation, and blunted hormonal signaling combine to quietly undermine vaccine efficacy in this population.

The immune system is a circadian organ. Internal clocks govern every aspect of immune function, from leukocyte trafficking to cytokine production and antibody generation. Sleep itself is an immune-modulatory state, optimizing the conditions necessary for the development of adaptive immunity. When shift work displaces sleep or fragments it across biologically inappropriate hours, the body's capacity to mount a robust immune response diminishes. It is not just the timing of sleep that matters, it is the timing of immune readiness.

Evidence for this disruption has been mounting. Recent research on hepatitis B vaccination outcomes in industrial shift workers revealed that those working rotating or night shifts were significantly more likely to fail to achieve a seroprotective response, despite receiving all three vaccine doses.[376] After adjusting for known confounders—age, sex, smoking status, and vitamin D levels—shift workers were three times more likely to remain non-responders compared to their day-working peers.[375] The finding was not due to missed appointments or incomplete dosing, but a biological failure to produce sufficient hepatitis B surface antibodies (HBsAb) after vaccination.

A handful of overlapping factors contribute to this failure. First is sleep disruption. Poor or inadequate sleep reduces natural killer cell activity, impairs antigen presentation, and alters cytokine expression.[377] Second is the hormonal impact of circadian misalignment. Elevated cortisol during the biological night, common among night shift workers, may suppress initial stages of vaccine-induced immunity.[378] Third is the high prevalence of vitamin D deficiency, a condition found in over 90% of shift workers in one cohort, which is known to impair B-cell and T-cell function and reduce antibody titers post-vaccination.[379]

Sex and age add further complexity. Male shift workers were especially at risk of vaccine nonresponse due to known sex differences in immune responsiveness.[376,377] Older age also correlated with poorer outcomes, a reminder that immunosenescence begins earlier when compounded by occupational stressors.

These findings extend beyond hepatitis B and apply to other vaccination responses as well. Past studies have shown that shift workers also demonstrate blunted responses to influenza and meningococcal vaccines.[377]

Sleep and circadian misalignment disrupt how the immune system recognizes, responds to, and remembers antigens, not through a vaccine-specific flaw, but through a systemic breakdown in biological timing. These insights demand a reevaluation of vaccination strategies for shift-working populations.

In an era of global outbreaks and vaccine-preventable illnesses, leaving a third of the workforce biologically unprotected is not just an oversight—it's a liability.

Until vaccination schedules reflect circadian biology, shift workers may remain biologically underprotected.

These are not just theoretical adjustments—they may become public health necessities, as ongoing research continues to shape our understanding. This recognition opens the door to a new kind of strategy: biologically attuned, circadian-aware, and grounded in the physiology of real people doing real work. Not only to protect individuals, but to safeguard the resilience of the systems they uphold.

Immune Alignment Protocol:

Optimizing Vaccine Response in Shift Workers, based on fixed schedules and uniform dosing, may not be enough. Instead, occupational health policies should consider:

- **Timing:** Administering vaccines during appropriate biological windows (e.g., early in the shift worker's "biological day") may enhance response.

- **Supplementation:** Screening and correcting vitamin D deficiency before vaccination could restore part of the immune deficit.

- **Booster Dosing:** Shift workers may benefit from tailored booster schedules or alternative vaccine formulations.

- **Recovery Periods:** Ensuring adequate sleep in the days following vaccination could improve antigen presentation and antibody production.

Metrics as a
Flashlight, Not a
Searchlight

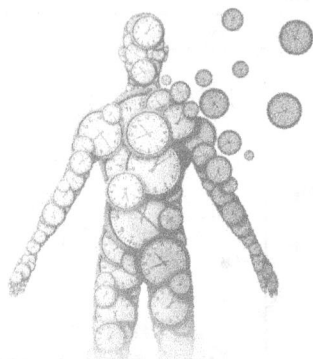

Your watch says you slept four hours. You feel fine. Who do you believe?

For the shift worker, one truth looms large: sleep is compromised. No algorithm is needed to confirm it. You don't need a wearable to prove what your body already knows.

Fatigue doesn't ask for permission. And recovery is elusive in a world that doesn't wait for rest.

Wearable health devices have exploded into our daily lives with the promise of empowerment. Marketed as tools to optimize sleep, track recovery, measure heart rate variability, and detect irregularities before symptoms arise, they seem like the perfect companion in the shift worker's fight against biological chaos.

But as with all tools, wearables cut both ways. Used well, they can foster insight. Used obsessively, they can fuel anxiety, confusion, and obsession with metrics that tell only part of the story.

For non-shift workers, believing you've had a bad night's sleep, based on faulty or misunderstood data, can sometimes make you *feel* worse, even when the sleep itself was sufficient. This phenomenon is well-documented: the power of suggestion is strong enough to alter cognition, mood, and performance. But shift workers don't need suggestion—they live in the trenches. When you wake up groggy after a short nap before your next shift, you're not questioning whether your tracker exaggerated the problem. You *feel* the problem.

For the shift worker, clarity matters: your device is a tool in your toolkit, not your boss. It should work for you, not rule over you.

Used wisely, wearables can provide invaluable feedback. For shift workers struggling to establish patterns amid rotating chaos, data can be a grounding force.

Tracking sleep duration can help uncover trends, like how consistent daytime sleep strategies or light-blocking curtains affect your rest. Monitoring resting heart rate or HRV (heart rate variability) can highlight how your body responds to caffeine, shift transitions, stress, or even a late-night meal.[380]

Devices that measure temperature and respiratory rate may offer early signs of illness, while blood oxygen tracking might reveal undiagnosed sleep apnea, common among night workers.[381,382]

For individuals with chronic health concerns, such as hypertension, atrial fibrillation, or diabetes, wearable monitoring can help capture meaningful trends.[383]

In fact, some shift workers credit their wearables for prompting life-saving early diagnoses. When used to enhance self-awareness, not control it, data becomes powerful.

But there is a darker side to data, especially when the numbers become the narrative. Enter orthosomnia: a newly recognized behavioral pattern where users become so fixated on getting "perfect sleep" that they actually develop insomnia.[384] It's sleep paralysis by obsession, where the fear of poor metrics hijacks the mind's ability to rest.

Sleep scientists first coined the term after seeing patients who were convinced their devices were more accurate than a full overnight sleep study. Some even requested prescription medication based solely on questionable tracker outputs, despite normal sleep confirmed in a lab.

This is not rare. For patients with heart rhythm disorders like atrial fibrillation (AFib), the issue is even more pronounced. A study published in the *Journal of the American Heart Association* found that wearable users with AFib were significantly more anxious, more likely to report symptoms, and more frequently contacted their healthcare teams, even when clinical confirmation of arrhythmia was absent.[385] One in five patients experienced intense fear from alerts that may or may not have been accurate.[384]

For night-shift workers already managing fatigue, these false alarms compound stress and erode confidence in their bodies.

This flood of anxiety drives up healthcare utilization, overburdens already strained systems, and, in some cases, worsens the very symptoms wearables were meant to monitor.

For those of us who work outside the rhythm of the sun, the truth is blunt: we are not chasing perfection. We are chasing sustainability. And in that pursuit, wearable data should be a flashlight, not a searchlight. It should illuminate patterns, not scrutinize every second of your night.

If your tracker tells you that you only slept 4 hours, but you feel capable and clear-headed, trust your body. If it reports "optimal recovery" but you can barely string thoughts together, believe your experience. No algorithm can capture your context: how long you've worked nights, whether you're juggling family obligations, if your hormones are shifting, or how your mental health is trending. Numbers are clean. Life is not.

For shift workers—especially nurses, paramedics, and first responders—metrics should inform, not dictate. The real value isn't in a single bad sleep score or a spike in heart rate. It's in the trends. The patterns. The quiet signals that emerge over time.

That's where the value is—not in the numbers themselves, but in what they help you notice. Metrics can't heal you. But they can guide you, if you let them illuminate your biology, not dictate it.

You are not a line graph. You are not your sleep score. You are a shift worker—resilient, adaptable, and fighting a battle most will never understand. And that makes you stronger than any wearable ever could. And that makes you more powerful than any wearable ever could.

Wearables are weather apps. They can predict, but they can't feel. You still have to step outside to face the storm.

Practical Advice: Keeping Wearables in Perspective

If you use a wearable, consider these principles:

Use trends, not snapshots. Weekly or monthly averages matter more than any one day.

Focus on what you can control. If sleep is limited, prioritize consistent timing, meal planning, and hydration.

Don't let bad data ruin a good day. Metrics are estimates—valuable, but fallible.

Track what matters most to you. If you feel stronger, more alert, or less irritable, that's meaningful, regardless of what your tracker says.

Use wearable insights to nudge behavior. If you learn that heavy meals hurt your sleep, change the habit, not your identity.

Neuroprotective
Gold

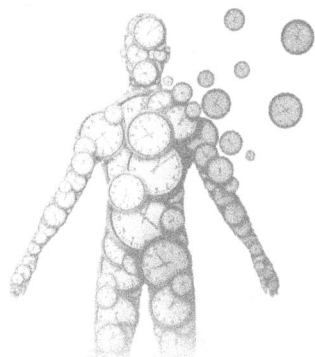

A physician I worked with once told me saffron was the first thing that helped her feel like herself again. Not high. Not numb. Just clear.

You won't find saffron in the vitamin aisle next to magnesium or fish oil.

It's not packaged in economy-sized capsules.

It's too expensive for that, too delicate, too storied.

Harvested by hand from the crocus flower, saffron's production is so labor-intensive that a single ounce can cost more than an ounce of silver.

Saffron is not here because it's trendy. It's here because it works, because it goes where fatigue lives and neurotransmitters falter. It belongs in the conversation about cognitive repair, not just general wellness. And for the modern shift worker, whose brain runs on cortisol, recycles sleep debt, and labors under chronic misalignment, saffron offers something rare: restoration.

We've walked through the foundations—omega-3s, PQQ, melatonin—the standard tools in the shift worker's survival kit. These are nutritional scaffolds, important, but limited. Saffron lives outside that framework. Not because it's exotic, but because its effects run deeper.

Saffron isn't listed alongside foundational compounds like magnesium or melatonin, not because it's less important, but because it's more specific, more advanced, and more expensive. It's not for everyone. But for those on the edge of cognitive exhaustion, navigating circadian strain and emotional depletion, saffron isn't just a supplement. It's a strategic intervention.

It deserves its own space because its mechanism is different. Its access is different. And its impact, for the right person, can be profound.

Saffron is what happens when ancient tradition meets molecular neuroscience. For centuries, it's been used in Persian and Ayurvedic medicine to elevate mood, sharpen focus, and calm an overstimulated mind.[386] Today, clinical studies are beginning to reveal the science behind the folklore.

This isn't hype. It's evidence. Saffron's bioactive compounds—crocin, crocetin, safranal, and picrocrocin—don't just flavor rice. They cross the blood-brain barrier.[386] They modulate neurotransmitters. They upregulate BDNF, a key protein involved in learning, memory, and neuroplasticity.[386] Saffron doesn't sedate like a benzodiazepine. It stabilizes. It fine-tunes. It returns the brain to a more adaptable baseline, especially in those who are sleep-deprived, emotionally overdrawn, or living on circadian credit.

Disrupted circadian rhythm changes more than your sleep schedule. It changes your brain. Blood flow decreases in prefrontal areas. Inflammatory cytokines rise. Executive function falters. Emotional regulation slips. You start losing yourself, not just in mood, but in identity. That's where saffron earns its place.

Studies have shown that saffron improves cerebral perfusion, enhancing oxygen delivery and nutrient flow to brain regions most affected by chronic stress and circadian misalignment.[387] In animal models of stroke and ischemia, saffron not only reduced infarct size but preserved neuron density in damaged cortical regions.[388]

Improved cerebral blood flow translates into sharper decision-making, better memory, and more stable mood—all under attack when your body's internal clock is out of sync with the sun. It also means more efficient detoxification through glymphatic flow, more ATP, and less brain fog.

Saffron's bioactive compounds act across multiple pathways, offering antioxidant protection, reducing inflammation, and supporting mitochondrial energy metabolism.[387]

Clinical trials in humans have shown improved mood scores and increased BDNF, an indicator of brain adaptability and recovery.[388] For shift workers experiencing chronic sleep loss, emotional fatigue, and executive function decline, these effects can mean the difference between burnout and balance.

Saffron has also been tested against SSRIs in the treatment of depression. In cases of mild to moderate symptoms, it has shown comparable effects, without the side effect burden.[389] That's critical for shift workers, especially in nursing, EMS, and night-shift caregiving, where pharmacologic options may feel too blunt, too risky, or too numbing.

One night-shift nurse shared:

"I didn't expect much. But after a few weeks, I felt sharper—not wired, just clearer. It was like my mind had more breathing room."

For those operating under cognitive strain and emotional depletion, saffron isn't a mood booster—it's a stabilizer.

A quiet recalibration. It's not a cure-all, but it's one of the few interventions that simultaneously supports mood, cognition, and cerebral blood flow. That makes it a triple threat in shift work medicine.

Saffron deserves its own chapter for the same reason red wine gets its own label: complexity, rarity, and depth. This isn't just something to try. It's an evidence-based tool, pharmacologically active, clinically studied, and culturally rooted. It exists at the intersection of food, medicine, and neuroprotection. For a population living outside the bounds of natural light and regular rest, that bridge matters.

Yes, saffron is expensive. It isn't mass-produced. It doesn't come in bulk. But neither does emotional resilience. Or mental clarity. Or the kind of neurobiological recovery shift workers desperately need. Saffron isn't a trend.

It's a strategy for clarity, resilience, and survival in a world that erodes them.

Supplement Protocol: Saffron

Form: Standardized saffron extract (e.g., 30 mg/day of crocin-containing product)

Timing: Take in the early evening on rest days; midday on shift days.

Duration: Clinical benefits often appear after 4–6 weeks of consistent use.

Onset: Subtle improvements in mood, clarity, or sleep may emerge within 2 weeks; full effects typically seen by 4–6 weeks.

Pairing: Combine with omega-3s for synergistic neurovascular effects.

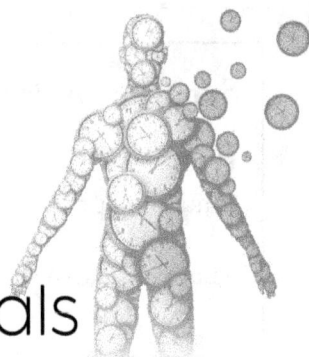

Reading the Signals

Before you go hunting for answers in your lab results, pause. This chapter is not about micromanaging your biology or turning bloodwork into a daily scoreboard. These numbers are not here to diagnose you in real time—they're here to reveal long-term trends. Patterns. Clues that emerge slowly, often before symptoms have a name. For shift workers, who live in a state of physiological distortion, these markers can serve as early warnings, not judgments. Not snapshots. But a quiet record of how your body is adapting to a life outside the 9-to-5.

Shift work changes how we eat, sleep, and recover, but it also changes something deeper: our biology. Beneath the surface, long before symptoms appear, your body begins to tell a story. A story most people never read. You don't have to guess at your health.

You can measure it. And in a world where chaos is normal and fatigue is expected, blood work becomes more than a wellness check—it becomes your early warning system.

This chapter isn't about turning you into a lab technician. It's about giving you the tools to recognize what matters. Because for the shift worker, knowledge isn't just power—it's protection.

You won't find these numbers on your fitness tracker. These are the deeper diagnostics, the lab markers that reflect stress, inflammation, nutrient status, and metabolic wear and tear.

They reveal what your schedule tries to hide. Subtle signals, not about crisis, but about course correction. Before we end, let's ground all this theory in the language your body already speaks: your blood.

Let's begin with one of the most disrupted signals in night-shift biology: vitamin D.

You work nights, spend your daylight hours asleep, or stay indoors under artificial light. That means your vitamin D levels are almost certainly low. And that matters more than you've been told.

Low vitamin D isn't just about weak bones; it's tied to low mood, impaired immune response, muscle fatigue, and a higher risk of metabolic syndrome.[390] For shift workers already burdened by immune and hormonal disruption, this deficiency adds fuel to the fire. Aim for a level between 40–60 ng/mL, and don't settle for "normal" if you're scraping the bottom of the reference range. Ask your provider for a 25(OH)D blood test and, if necessary, supplement with D3 + K2, ideally taken in the morning or mid-day to support your natural rhythm.[391]

Then there's hemoglobin A1c, your three-month glucose report card. Glucose doesn't lie, and neither does your A1c. It reflects your average blood sugar over the past 8–12 weeks. For shift workers who skip meals, snack at odd hours, or rely on quick carbs to survive night shifts, this number often creeps up silently. Elevated A1c isn't just about diabetes—it predicts cognitive decline, fatigue, and inflammation.[392] Ideally, your A1c should stay below 5.6%.[391] If it trends upward, reconsider your night meals, adopt time-restricted eating on off days, and talk to your provider about early intervention.

High-sensitivity C-reactive protein, or hs-CRP, is your internal inflammation alarm. This marker doesn't diagnose a disease—it reveals a state. A chronically elevated hs-CRP means your body is fighting something, even if you feel "fine."[393] Shift workers, with their disrupted sleep, chronic stress, and metabolic strain, are prone to this type of silent inflammation. Keep your hs-CRP below 1.0 mg/L. If it's higher, it's time to double down on sleep quality, omega-3 intake, and anti-inflammatory nutrition.

Next is your thyroid, the metabolism triad: TSH, free T3, and free T4. These hormones regulate your energy, focus, temperature, and weight.[394] And because the thyroid axis is sensitive to circadian disruption, shift work can push it out of balance. Especially in women, even small deviations can create big problems: fatigue, anxiety, low mood, and weight changes.[393]

Aim for a TSH between 0.5–2.5 mIU/L, and make sure you ask for a full thyroid panel. If your results are technically "normal" but you still feel off, don't dismiss your symptoms—insist on deeper testing.

Ferritin is your iron storage marker, but its relevance goes far beyond anemia. Low ferritin, even within the "normal" range, can cause brain fog, shortness of breath, and exhaustion, especially for menstruating individuals or anyone with disrupted sleep architecture.[395,396]

An optimal range is 50–100 ng/mL.[395] If you're under that threshold, consider iron-rich foods or supplementation, paired with vitamin C for absorption. Recheck every 3–6 months until you stabilize.

But iron isn't the only nutrient that matters. Two others, vitamin B12 and folate, often slip under the radar but quietly erode cognitive function when overlooked.

Low B12 is especially common in those who take acid blockers, follow plant-based diets, or live with chronic stress (sound familiar?).[397] Aim for a B12 level between 500–900 pg/mL.[396] Symptoms like fatigue, tingling, or memory lapses can appear even when you're technically "within range." [396] If supplementation is needed, look for methylated forms such as methylcobalamin, which are more readily absorbed.

These aren't exotic markers. They're the basics, the quiet signals shift workers often overlook.

So what do you do with all of this?

Here's the bigger picture: blood doesn't lie, but it doesn't tell the whole story. Labs are tools, not truths. Just like wearables, they must be interpreted in context.

Your A1c doesn't measure your willpower. A low vitamin D level doesn't mean you failed. Your body is a dynamic, adaptive system, not a spreadsheet. But when labs are tracked over time, they become something more: a map. A personalized blueprint that helps you recover, adapt, and course-correct before symptoms scream louder than the data.

This matters because shift work isn't just exhausting—it's biologically distorting. Your internal clocks fall out of sync with the natural world. That mismatch creates biochemical stress. Blood tests help you catch the damage before it becomes disease. By monitoring the right markers, you create feedback loops. You learn what foods help. What sleep routines heal. What supplements restore. You shift from guessing to knowing. From surviving to adapting. From defense to offense.

That shift starts with action—measurable, repeatable action. If you've never had a comprehensive blood panel, start now. Keep a copy. Track your numbers. Share them with your provider. And don't accept "you're within range" if your body says otherwise. Normal isn't always optimal. And optimal isn't static—it's personal. Because in a world where shift workers give their best to everyone else, your health deserves more than guesswork. It deserves numbers. It deserves context. And it deserves care.

Let your labs be a flashlight, not a searchlight. You just need enough light to see where you're going, and when to course-correct. This isn't about chasing perfection. It's about resilience, the quiet ability to adapt before the damage becomes disease.

Epilogue:
The Rhythm You
Still Carry

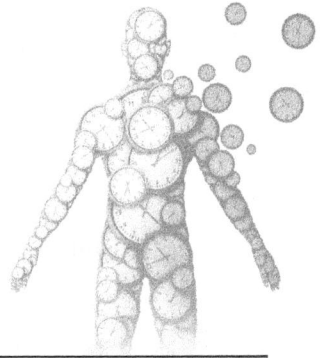

You weren't designed for this schedule. Your biology didn't evolve under fluorescent lights, on fractured sleep, or with cortisol as your co-pilot. And yet, here you are.

You've adapted. Improvised. Shown up. Again and again.

This book wasn't written to glorify that grind. It was written to honor the cost of it, and to give you a way back to center. Because shift work is not just a job. It's a physiologic gamble. A cognitive drain. An emotional tax. And for many of us, a calling.

You carry the weight of critical hours. You hold the line in the silence while the rest of the world sleeps. And often, you do it invisibly.

But your body keeps score, even when no one else does.

That's the paradox: you can be essential and unseen. Skilled and exhausted. Strong and biologically off-track.

So if you take one thing from this book, let it be this: You are not broken. You are misaligned. And misalignment is not a flaw—it's a solvable mismatch.

You've now seen the science. You've read the signs in your blood, your sleep, your hunger, your mood. It's not about rigid routines—it's about reclaiming rhythm, one shift at a time.

You deserve a biology that serves you. You deserve clarity. Recovery. Agency.

Because the system may not have been built for you, but that doesn't mean you can't build within it.

The rhythm is still there. Under the caffeine, under the night lights, under the exhaustion. It's quiet, but waiting.

And you? You're not just surviving. You're realigning.

Thank you for showing up—on the job, and for yourself. Unseen by many, essential to all.

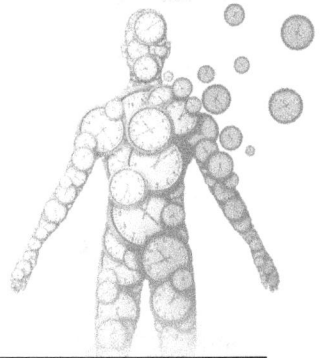

Appendix

APPENDIX A: YOUR RHYTHM™ GUIDE TO SHIFT WORK HEALTH

R = Restorative Sleep

Prioritize both quantity and quality. Use blackout curtains, melatonin (when needed), and consistent pre-/post-shift routines to help recalibrate your circadian system, even when you're working against it.

H = Hydration & Nutrition

Stay hydrated and time meals strategically. Avoid high-sugar or ultra-processed foods during night shifts. Emphasize time-restricted eating and prioritize fueling during your biological "day", even if it falls at night.

Y = You-Centered Movement

Exercise for adaptation, not aesthetics. Incorporate HIIT and post-shift movement to support metabolic health, mental clarity, and circadian alignment.

T = Track & Test

Know your numbers. From vitamin D and ferritin to A1c and CRP, bloodwork offers early warning. Use wearables to spot trends, not to define your worth.

H = Hormonal & Mental Health

Understand how shift work disrupts cortisol, melatonin, and insulin cycles. Support emotional resilience through adaptogens like ashwagandha, saffron, or professional care when needed.

M = Manage Light & Misalignment

Use light exposure like a prescription. Seek bright light before night shifts, block blue light after. Circadian misalignment isn't a failure—it's a mismatch that demands active countermeasures.

APPENDIX B: FOUNDATIONAL SUPPLEMENT SCHEDULE – NIGHT SHIFT BLOCK (TUES–THURS)

Monday (Pre-shift prep & circadian stabilization)

Goal: Build biological stability and prep for transition

- 9:00 a.m. – Vitamin D3 (2,000 IU) + B-complex (25–50 mg)

- 12:00 p.m. – Omega-3 (1,000 mg EPA/DHA)

- 6:00 p.m. – Magnesium glycinate (300 mg)

- 9:00 p.m. – L-theanine (200 mg)

- *Optional:* L-tryptophan (1g) if sleep latency is high

Tuesday (First night shift)

Goal: Promote alertness; protect post-shift sleep

Pre Shift

- 4:00 p.m. – Vitamin D3 + B-complex

- 5:30 p.m. – Omega-3

- 6:30 p.m. – Caffeine (100–200 mg) + L-theanine (100 mg)

Post Shift

- 8:00 a.m. – Magnesium glycinate

- 9:00 a.m. – L-theanine (200 mg)

- 9:30 a.m. – Melatonin (0.5–1 mg)

- *Optional:* L-ornithine (400 mg) to blunt cortisol

Wednesday (Second night shift)

Goal: Sustain rhythm, support cognition and recovery

Pre Shift

- 4:00 p.m. – Vitamin D3 + B-complex

- 5:30 p.m. – Omega-3

- 6:30 p.m. – Caffeine + L-theanine

Post Shift

- 8:00 a.m. – Magnesium glycinate

- 9:00 a.m. – L-theanine

- 9:30 a.m. – Melatonin

- *Optional:* Ashwagandha (300 mg KSM-66) upon waking

Thursday (Final night shift)

Goal: Support final alert period + begin shift-back strategy

Pre Shift

- 4:00 p.m. – Vitamin D3 + B-complex

- 5:30 p.m. – Omega-3

- 6:30 p.m. – Caffeine + L-theanine

Post Shift

- 8:00 a.m. – Magnesium glycinate

- 9:00 a.m. – L-theanine

- 9:30 a.m. – Melatonin (optional if adjusting schedule)

- 9:30 a.m. – *Add:* L-serine (3g) if using bright light Friday morning

Friday (Transition day)
Goal: Begin circadian re-entrainment

- Post-shift nap (90 minutes)

- 10:00 a.m. – Vitamin D3 + omega-3

- 11:00 a.m. – Bright light exposure + L-serine (3g)

- 6:00 p.m. – Magnesium glycinate

- 9:00 p.m. – L-theanine

- *Avoid melatonin unless sleeping during the day again*

Saturday (Daytime recovery)
Goal: Stabilize circadian rhythm and reduce inflammation

- 9:00 a.m. – Vitamin D3 + B-complex

- 12:00 p.m. – Omega-3

- 6:00 p.m. – Magnesium glycinate

- 9:00 p.m. – L-theanine

- *Optional:* Apigenin (50 mg) for sleep support

Sunday (Reset & prep for week ahead)
Goal: Maintain alignment, prep for shift cycle

- 9:00 a.m. – Vitamin D3 + omega-3

- 12:00 p.m. – Light exposure, hydration, movement

- 6:00 p.m. – Magnesium glycinate\

- 9:00 p.m. – L-theanine

- *Optional:* L-tryptophan (1g) if prepping for early sleep

APPENDIX C: TARGETED SUPPLEMENT SCHEDULE – NIGHT SHIFT BLOCK (TUES–THURS)

Monday (Stabilization + pre-shift readiness)

Goal: Prime neurotransmitter balance and recovery systems

- 9:00 a.m. – CDP-choline (250–500 mg) for cognitive support

- 12:00 p.m. – Rhodiola rosea (200–400 mg) to buffer fatigue

- 6:00 p.m. – Apigenin (50 mg) for circadian wind-down

- 9:00 p.m. – L-theanine (200 mg) + glycine (3g) before sleep

- Optional: PEA (350 mg) for sleep latency support

Tuesday (First night shift)

Goal: Support alertness and post-shift sleep recovery

Pre Shift

- 4:00 p.m. – CDP-choline (500 mg) + acetyl-L-carnitine (1,000 mg)

- 5:30 p.m. – Rhodiola (200 mg) + omega-3s (if used alongside, 2–3g)

- 6:30 p.m. – Caffeine (100–200 mg) + L-theanine (100 mg)

Post Shift

- 8:00 a.m. (post-shift) – Magnesium glycinate (300 mg if tolerated)

- 9:00 a.m. – Apigenin (50 mg) + L-theanine (200 mg)

- 9:30 a.m. – Melatonin (0.5–1 mg) + PEA (350 mg) before sleep

Wednesday (Second night shift)
Goal: Sustain neurocognitive function and manage fatigue
Pre Shift
- 4:00 p.m. – CDP-choline (250 mg) + lion's mane (500–1,000 mg)
- 5:30 p.m. – Rhodiola (200–400 mg) + acetyl-L-carnitine
- 6:30 p.m. – Caffeine + L-theanine

Post Shift
- 8:00 a.m. – Astaxanthin (6–12 mg) for neuroimmune protection
- 9:00 a.m. – Apigenin + glycine
- 9:30 a.m. – Melatonin + PEA

Thursday (Final night shift)
Goal: Transition support + protect cognitive clarity
Pre Shift
- 4:00 p.m. – Ashwagandha (Shoden® 120–240 mg or KSM-66® 300 mg)
- 5:30 p.m. – Lion's mane + rhodiola
- 6:30 p.m. – Caffeine + L-theanine

Post Shift
- 8:00 a.m. – CoQ10 (100–300 mg) + PQQ (10–20 mg)
- 9:00 a.m. – Apigenin + glycine
- 9:30 a.m. – Melatonin (if continuing night rhythm)
- Optional: L-serine (3g) before morning light to phase-shift circadian rhythm

Friday (Shift-back and circadian realignment)

Goal: Reset internal rhythm and support neuroprotection

- Post-shift nap (90 min) — then proceed

- 10:00 a.m. – PQQ + CoQ10 with breakfast

- 11:00 a.m. – Bright light therapy + L-serine (3g)\

- 6:00 p.m. – Ashwagandha or apigenin for evening calm

- 9:00 p.m. – L-theanine + PEA + glycine

- Avoid melatonin unless continuing night sleep pattern

Saturday (Deep recovery and mood stabilization)

Goal: Cellular regeneration + stress modulation

- 9:00 a.m. – Lion's mane + rhodiola

- 12:00 p.m. – CDP-choline for mental clarity

- 6:00 p.m. – Apigenin

- 9:00 p.m. – L-theanine + PEA before bed

Sunday (Recalibrate & prep week ahead)

Goal: Maintain sleep integrity and cognitive readiness

- 9:00 a.m. – Astaxanthin or NAC for antioxidant support

- 12:00 p.m. – CoQ10 + CDP-choline

- 6:00 p.m. – Ashwagandha

- 9:00 p.m. – Apigenin + glycine + L-theanine

Summary of Transition Day Schedule (e.g., Friday)

Note: While this plan uses Friday as an example, your personal transition day may fall on a different day of the week depending on your shift rotation. The principles remain the same; this is about resetting your circadian rhythm from night shift misalignment back to a daytime schedule.

Morning: Anchor nap approach—sleep a few hours after your last night shift (2–4 hrs.), then push through the day until early bedtime.

Take vitamin D3 and omega-3s with breakfast to reinforce morning signals. At ~11:00 a.m., get bright light exposure and take 3g of L-serine to jump-start your circadian phase shift. Stay awake and active after this point—no going back to bed.

Afternoon: No planned naps unless absolutely necessary. Use light exposure, mild exercise, and hydration to stay alert. Caffeine can help, but avoid it after early afternoon. The goal here is to stretch your waking window just enough to build healthy sleep pressure by evening. You're using light, movement, and strategic supplements to push through the day, so your body is ready to sleep at the right time.

Evening: Take magnesium around 6:00 p.m. to initiate your wind-down. At 9:00 p.m., take glycine and L-theanine to promote relaxation and lower core body temperature. Begin dimming lights and avoiding screens to support melatonin rise and signal that bedtime is near.

Night: Be in bed by 9:30–10:00 p.m. Aim for 7–9 hours of sleep. This marks your official reentry into a day-oriented cycle. If the plan works, you'll wake up Saturday morning more aligned, closer to the rhythm your biology prefers.

Why It Matters

This (e.g., Friday) is your transition day. Its purpose isn't just recovery—it's circadian re-entrainment. Every cue—light, supplements, meal timing, and activity—is designed to nudge your internal clock back into sync with the outside world. And that shift doesn't happen in theory—it happens when you sleep.

This approach isn't about perfection. It's about traction. Friday night sleep isn't just rest—it's your re-entry into rhythm. A small step, but the first toward resilience in a life lived out of sync.

APPENDIX D: PRECISION RX MODAFINIL (PROVIGIL®)

Precision Alertness Protocol: Modafinil (Provigil®)

Purpose: Sustain cognitive performance and vigilance on night shifts while minimizing sleep disruption and supporting circadian resilience.

Monday (Pre-shift prep & stabilization)

Goal: No modafinil, protect baseline sleep physiology

- **No modafinil recommended**

- *Focus:* Circadian preparation through consistent light cues, magnesium, and wind-down routine

Tuesday (First night shift)

Goal: Support alertness onset and performance across the night

- **6:00 p.m. (1 hour before shift) – Modafinil 100–200 mg**

  o Start with 100 mg if first-time use or sensitive to stimulants

  o Take with a small snack and water

  o Avoid redosing

Wednesday (Second night shift)

Goal: Sustain neurocognitive performance without residual stimulation

- **6:00 p.m. – Modafinil 100–200 mg**

  o If prior night's recovery sleep was reduced, consider lowering dose

  o Maintain hydration and avoid caffeine layering

Thursday (Final night shift)

Goal: Optional use based on fatigue level and post-shift sleep needs

- **6:00 p.m. – Modafinil 100 mg (optional)**
  - If transitioning back to daytime rhythm Friday, skip or halve dose
  - Prioritize post-shift sleep quality over last-shift productivity

Friday (Transition day)

Goal: Begin circadian re-entrainment

- **No modafinil recommended**
- *Instead:* Post-shift nap (~90 min), bright light exposure by 11:00 a.m., movement, hydration

Saturday & Sunday (Recovery & reset)

Goal: Support circadian normalization and neurochemical reset

- No modafinil
- *Supportive cues:* Natural morning light, consistent wake time, no stimulants after noon

Key Usage Guidelines

- **Timing:** Take modafinil **exactly 1 hour before scheduled shift start**
- **Dosing:** 100–200 mg once daily; do not exceed 200 mg in 24 hours
- **Sleep hygiene matters:** Avoid caffeine late in shift; protect sleep environment post-shift
- **Strategic use only:** Reserve for high-demand blocks; do not use continuously or outside of shift work

APPENDIX E: PRECISION RX ARMODAFINIL (NUVIGIL®)

Purpose: Enhance alertness with longer duration of action while minimizing early morning fatigue during extended shifts.

Monday (Baseline)

Goal: Establish natural sleep without pharmacologic stimulation

- No armodafinil recommended

- Prioritize baseline circadian cues (light, magnesium, structured sleep timing)

Tuesday (First night shift)

Goal: Initiate long-duration alertness with reduced early-morning crash

- 6:00 p.m. – Armodafinil 150 mg

  o Take with water 1 hour before shift

  o Avoid redosing or stacking with caffeine late in shift

Wednesday (Second night shift)

Goal: Maintain wakefulness without sleep compromise

- 6:00 p.m. – Armodafinil 150 mg

  o Adjust downward (100 mg) if post-shift sleep quality was poor

Thursday (Final night shift)

Goal: Optional use to support final shift performance

- 6:00 p.m. – Armodafinil 100 mg (optional)

  o If planning circadian reset Friday, consider skipping dose

Friday–Sunday (Recovery & realignment)

Goal: Sleep restoration and rhythm reset

- No armodafinil recommended

- Focus: Light cues, sleep hygiene, recovery supplements

Usage Notes:
- Longer half-life (~15 hours) than modafinil—plan sleep accordingly
- Less "wear-off" fatigue but higher potential for sleep onset delays if used late
- Do not use on back-to-back recovery days to preserve sleep quality

APPENDIX F: PRECISION RX SOLRIAMFETOL (SUNOSI®)

Purpose: Support wakefulness in late-shift hours when other agents wear off; ideal for those who need longer, more stable stimulant support.

Tuesday–Thursday (Night shifts)
- 6:00 p.m. – Solriamfetol 75–150 mg
- Start with 75 mg; increase only if no adverse cardiovascular symptoms
- Avoid additional stimulants; maintain hydration
- Monitor for blood pressure and heart rate increases

Friday–Sunday
- No solriamfetol recommended
- Focus: Restore sleep integrity; avoid residual stimulation

Usage Notes:
- Dual norepinephrine/dopamine reuptake inhibitor
- Rapid onset; long half-life (~6–8 hours) supports early morning alertness

- May interfere with post-shift sleep—use only when prolonged wakefulness is necessary
- Contraindicated in uncontrolled hypertension or arrhythmia history

APPENDIX G: CHRONOTYPE QUIZ FOR SHIFT WORKERS

Purpose: This quiz helps shift workers identify their natural chronotype—Morning Type (Lark), Evening Type (Owl), or Intermediate Type (Hummingbird)—even with irregular schedules.

Instructions: Answer based on how you feel on days off or when you're not influenced by your shift schedule. Each answer corresponds to a point value. Tally your total at the end.

1. On days off, what time do you naturally wake up (without an alarm)?

A. Before 7:00 AM

B. After 10:00 AM

C. Between 7:00 and 9:30 AM

2. How do you feel when starting a day shift (e.g., 7:00 AM start)?

A. Energized and clear-headed

B. Extremely tired and foggy

C. I can manage, but I need time to adjust

3. How do you adapt to night shifts (e.g., 7:00 PM–7:00 AM)?

A. I struggle to stay awake and alert

B. I feel productive and sharp through the night

C. It's challenging, but I can adjust over time

4. On your first day off after a night shift, what do you do?

A. Go to bed early to reset to daytime

B. Stay up late or sleep in late—it feels natural

C. Take a nap and gradually return to a daytime routine

5. When do you prefer to exercise on days off?

A. Early morning

B. Late evening or nighttime

C. Midday or early evening

6. What best describes your cognitive function in the evening (after 6:00 PM)?

A. I'm winding down and feeling tired

B. I'm most focused and mentally sharp

C. I'm functional, but not at peak performance

7. How easy is it for you to fall asleep after a night shift?

A. Very difficult—I feel out of sync

B. Pretty easy—I'm tired and used to it

C. Somewhat difficult, but sleep routines (or, if advised by a clinician, melatonin) help

Scoring System: A = 3 points (Morning preference) B = 1 point (Evening preference) C = 2 points (Intermediate preference)

Score Range: 7–21

Interpretation

- **17–21: Morning Type (Lark)** – Naturally alert early; structured routines suit you.

- **12–16: Intermediate Type (Hummingbird)** – Adaptable; function well across schedules.

- **7–11: Evening Type (Owl)** – More alert later; may handle nights more easily.

Example: Q1 A(3) + Q2 C(2) + Q3 B(1) + Q4 B(1) + Q5 C(2) + Q6 A(3) + Q7 C(2) = **14 → Intermediate (Hummingbird)**

Tips by Chronotype

Morning Type

- Prioritize morning or early shifts
- Use bright light soon after waking
- Avoid caffeine later in the day

Evening Type

- Night/evening shifts may fit better
- Watch for accumulating sleep debt
- Use blackout curtains and a consistent wind-down

Intermediate Type

- Rotate shifts gradually when possible
- Keep sleep and wake times as consistent as you can
- Optimize light exposure (bright light on wake; dim light before sleep)

Note: This is an educational self-screen, not a diagnostic tool. Chronotype can be influenced by light exposure, social schedules, and health factors. For persistent sleep issues or to use melatonin safely, consult a qualified clinician.

Glossary of Terms

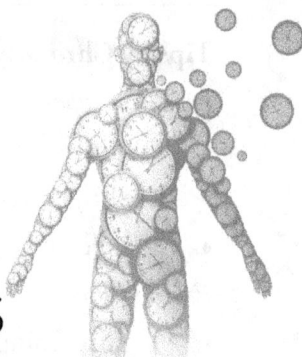

ADORA2A – A gene encoding the adenosine A2A receptor, which influences sleep regulation, arousal, and caffeine sensitivity.

ADRB1 – A gene encoding the beta-1 adrenergic receptor, involved in cardiovascular regulation and circadian rhythm entrainment.

A1c (Hemoglobin A1c) – A biomarker reflecting average blood glucose over the past 2–3 months; used to diagnose and monitor diabetes.

ACTH (Adrenocorticotropic Hormone) – A pituitary hormone that stimulates cortisol release from the adrenal glands.

Actigraphy – A method of measuring rest-activity cycles using motion sensors, often via wearable devices.

Adaptogens – Natural substances (e.g., ashwagandha, rhodiola) that enhance resilience to physical and mental stress.

AFib (Atrial Fibrillation) – A cardiac arrhythmia characterized by irregular, rapid heartbeats, associated with fatigue and cardiovascular risk.

ALCAR (Acetyl-L-Carnitine) – A mitochondrial nutrient and supplement that supports energy production and cognitive function.

ALT (Alanine Aminotransferase) – A liver enzyme measured in blood tests; elevated levels may indicate liver dysfunction.

AMPK (AMP-Activated Protein Kinase) – A cellular energy sensor that regulates metabolism, influenced by circadian rhythms and exercise.

Armodafinil – A wakefulness-promoting medication prescribed for Shift Work Sleep Disorder and narcolepsy; the R-enantiomer of modafinil.

Ashwagandha – An adaptogenic herb (Withania somnifera) shown to reduce stress, improve sleep quality, and support hormonal balance.

AST (Aspartate Aminotransferase) – A liver enzyme; elevated levels may indicate muscle or liver injury.

ATP (Adenosine Triphosphate) – The primary cellular energy currency, produced in mitochondria and critical for muscle and brain function.

Caffeine – A central nervous system stimulant that blocks adenosine receptors, promoting alertness and delaying fatigue.

Cancer – A group of diseases marked by uncontrolled cell growth; night shift work is classified as a probable carcinogen due to circadian disruption.

Chrononutrition – The study of how the timing of food intake affects circadian rhythms, metabolism, and overall health.

Chronotype – An individual's natural sleep-wake preference, ranging from early ("morning larks") to late ("night owls").

Circadian Rhythm – The internal biological cycle (~24 hours) that regulates sleep, metabolism, hormones, and alertness.

Coenzyme Q10 (CoQ10) – A mitochondrial antioxidant and cofactor in energy production; used as a dietary supplement for fatigue and cardiovascular health.

Cortisol – A glucocorticoid hormone involved in stress response, metabolism, and circadian rhythm; normally peaks in the morning.

CRP (C-Reactive Protein) – A biomarker of inflammation measured in blood tests; elevated levels indicate systemic stress or disease.

Diabetes Mellitus Type 2 – A metabolic disorder marked by insulin resistance and chronic hyperglycemia, associated with shift work and circadian misalignment.

Dopamine – A neurotransmitter regulating reward, motivation, movement, and alertness; sensitive to sleep loss and stimulants.

Ferritin – A blood protein that stores iron; low levels are associated with anemia and fatigue.

FSH (Follicle-Stimulating Hormone) – A reproductive hormone that regulates ovarian follicle development and spermatogenesis.

Ghrelin – A stomach-derived hormone that stimulates appetite; levels rise with sleep deprivation and energy restriction.

Growth Hormone (GH) – A hormone released during deep sleep that supports tissue repair, metabolism, and muscle health.

Insulin – A hormone secreted by the pancreas that regulates glucose uptake and blood sugar levels.

Insulin Resistance – A condition in which cells respond poorly to insulin, leading to elevated blood glucose and metabolic dysfunction.

Leptin – A hormone secreted by fat cells that signals satiety and regulates energy balance; levels fall with sleep restriction.

LH (Luteinizing Hormone) – A pituitary hormone that triggers ovulation and regulates testosterone production.

Magnesium – A mineral essential for muscle, nerve, and circadian function; often used as a supplement for sleep quality.

Melatonin – A hormone secreted by the pineal gland at night, signaling the body to prepare for sleep.

Metabolic Syndrome – A cluster of conditions—including central obesity, hypertension, high blood sugar, and abnormal cholesterol—that increase cardiovascular risk.

Methylphenidate – A central nervous system stimulant that increases dopamine and norepinephrine levels; used to treat ADHD and sometimes fatigue.

Modafinil – A wakefulness-promoting medication approved for Shift Work Sleep Disorder and narcolepsy.

N-Acetylcysteine (NAC) – A precursor to glutathione with antioxidant properties, used to reduce oxidative stress.

Neurodegeneration – The progressive loss of neurons and brain function, seen in conditions such as Alzheimer's and Parkinson's disease.

Neuroplasticity – The brain's capacity to adapt structurally and functionally in response to experience, learning, and recovery.

Neuroprotection – Strategies, compounds, or interventions that preserve brain function and protect against injury.

PCOS (Polycystic Ovarian Syndrome) – A hormonal-metabolic disorder characterized by irregular cycles, hyperandrogenism, and insulin resistance.

Perimenopause – The transitional period before menopause marked by fluctuating hormone levels and irregular cycles.

Pitolisant – A histamine-3 receptor antagonist used to promote wakefulness in narcolepsy and studied in shift work fatigue.

Polysomnography – A diagnostic sleep study that records brain waves, oxygen levels, breathing, and sleep stages.

Postprandial Glucose – Blood sugar concentration measured after meals; typically elevated when meals are eaten late at night.

PQQ (Pyrroloquinoline Quinone) – A redox cofactor that supports mitochondrial health, antioxidant defense, and neuroprotection.

Progesterone – A reproductive hormone essential for menstrual cycle regulation and pregnancy maintenance.

Recovery Sleep – Sleep obtained after deprivation or restriction, often longer and deeper than baseline sleep.

Resilience – The capacity to adapt and maintain function despite stressors such as sleep loss or circadian disruption.

Serotonin – A neurotransmitter involved in mood, appetite, and sleep regulation; a precursor to melatonin.

Shift Work Sleep Disorder (SWSD) – A circadian rhythm disorder marked by insomnia, excessive sleepiness, and impaired performance due to misaligned work schedules.

Sirtuins – A family of proteins that regulate metabolism, aging, and circadian processes.

Sleep Hygiene – A set of practices and environmental conditions that promote high-quality, restorative sleep.

Sleep Inertia – The grogginess and impaired performance experienced immediately upon waking.

Solriamfetol – A dopamine and norepinephrine reuptake inhibitor used to treat excessive sleepiness in shift work sleep disorder.

Suprachiasmatic Nucleus (SCN) – The brain's master circadian clock, located in the hypothalamus.

Testosterone – A hormone involved in male reproductive function, muscle mass, and energy regulation; sensitive to sleep loss.

Theobromine – A naturally occurring stimulant found in cocoa, structurally similar to caffeine but with milder effects.

Time-Restricted Eating (TRE) – A dietary pattern in which eating is confined to a daily time window, aligning metabolism with circadian rhythms.

Vitamin D – A fat-soluble vitamin important for bone health, immunity, and circadian regulation; often supplemented in shift workers.

Wearables – Digital devices (e.g., smartwatches, rings) that track sleep, activity, and physiological markers.

Work-Span Health – The long-term trajectory of health and performance across a working career.

Zeitgeber – An external environmental cue, such as light, food, or activity, that synchronizes circadian rhythms to the day-night cycle.

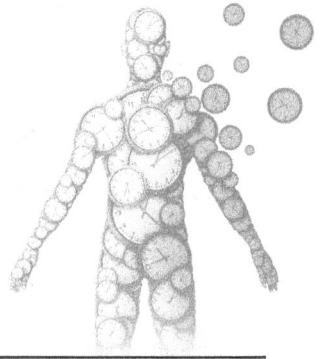

Endnotes

The Hard Truth

1 WNEP. (2013, November 5). *Critical care doctor tries to save woman after crash in Northumberland County.* WNEP. https://www.wnep.com/article/news/local/northumberland-county/critical-care-doctor-tries-to-save-woman-after-crash-in-northumberland-county/523-39fe5bbe-f8e9-4fbe-aa46-0bf22b4e5e5e

2 Fox 5 Atlanta. (2025, March 25). *Forsyth County nurse claims she fell asleep before fatal crash on Highway 9.* Fox 5 Atlanta. https://www.fox5atlanta.com/news/forsyth-county-nurse-claims-she-fell-asleep-before-fatal-crash-highway-9

3 Tefft, B. C. (2014). *Prevalence of Motor Vehicle Crashes Involving Drowsy Drivers, United States, 2009–2013.* AAA Foundation for Traffic Safety. https://aaafoundation.org/prevalence-drowsy-driving-crashes/

4 Lee, M. L., Howard, M. E., Horrey, W. J., Liang, Y., Anderson, C., Rajaratnam, S. M. W., & Czeisler, C. A. (2016). High risk of near-crash driving events following night-shift work. *Proceedings of the National Academy of Sciences of the United States of America, 113*(1), 176–181. https://doi.org/10.1073/pnas.1510383112

The Biological Price Tag

5 U.S. Bureau of Labor Statistics. (2020). *Workers on flexible and shift schedules in 2017–2018.* Retrieved from https://www.bls.gov/news.release/flex2.nr0.htm

6 American Academy of Sleep Medicine. (2014). *International classification of sleep disorders* (3rd ed.).

7   International Agency for Research on Cancer (IARC). (2024). *List of Classifications – IARC Monographs Volumes 1–135.* Retrieved from https://monographs.iarc.who.int/list-of-classifications/

8   Munteanu, C., Turti, S., Achim, L., Muresan, R., Souca, M., Prifti, E., Mârza, S. M., & Papuc, I. (2024). The Relationship between Circadian Rhythm and Cancer Disease. *International journal of molecular sciences, 25*(11), 5846. https://doi.org/10.3390/ijms25115846

9   Kecklund, G., & Axelsson, J. (2016). Health consequences of shift work and insufficient sleep. *BMJ*, 355, i5210. https://doi.org/10.1136/bmj.i5210

Ancient Rhythms and Contemporary Challenges

10 Alcantara, J. (2018, May 8). *The Firefighters of Ancient Rome.* Ancient History Blog – City of Rome. Macquarie University. Retrieved July 10, 2025, from https://ancient-history-blog.mq.edu.au/cityOfRome/Vigiles

11 Craig, R. P. (2019). *The industrial revolution in world history* (5th ed.). Routledge. https://doi.org/10.4324/9780429494475

12 Dublin, T. (1993). *Women at work: The transformation of work and community in Lowell, Massachusetts, 1826–1860.* Columbia University Press. https://hdl.handle.net/2027/heb00092.0001.001

13 U.S. Bureau of Labor Statistics. (2023). *Employed persons working shift schedules by occupation and industry* [Table 18]. U.S. Department of Labor. https://www.bls.gov/cps/cpsaat18.htm

14 Redline. (2024). *Shift work statistics: How it affects health, sleep, and performance.* https://redline.digital/shift-work-statistic

15 Kecklund, G., & Axelsson, J. (2016). Health consequences of shift work and insufficient sleep. *BMJ (Clinical research ed.),* 355, i5210. https://doi.org/10.1136/bmj.i5210

16 Reinganum, M. I., & Thomas, J. (2024, February 12). *Shift work hazards.* In StatPearls. StatPearls Publishing. https://www.ncbi.nlm.nih.gov/books/NBK589670/

17 Malik, V., Huang, X., Zhou, H., Bojar, R., Soni, R. K., Landry, D. W., Jelic, S., & Wang, J. (2025). Multiomics reveal biomolecular shifts and ER stress in sleep-restricted women affecting NSC functions. *iScience*, *28*(5), 112510. https://doi.org/10.1016/j.isci.2025.112510

18 Freiberg A. S. (2020). Why We Sleep: A Hypothesis for an Ultimate or Evolutionary Origin for Sleep and Other Physiological Rhythms. *Journal of circadian rhythms*, *18*, 2. https://doi.org/10.5334/jcr.189

Our Biochemical Pacemaker

19 Panda S. (2016). Circadian physiology of metabolism. *Science (New York, N.Y.)*, *354*(6315), 1008–1015. https://doi.org/10.1126/science.aah4967

20 Bass, J., & Lazar, M. A. (2016). Circadian time signatures of fitness and disease. *Science (New York, N.Y.)*, *354*(6315), 994–999. https://doi.org/10.1126/science.aah4965

21 Ma, M. A., & Morrison, E. H. (2023, July 24). Neuroanatomy, nucleus suprachiasmatic. In StatPearls. StatPearls Publishing. https://www.ncbi.nlm.nih.gov/books/NBK546664/

22 Paul, K. N., Saafir, T. B., & Tosini, G. (2009). The role of retinal photoreceptors in the regulation of circadian rhythms. *Reviews in endocrine & metabolic disorders*, *10*(4), 271–278. https://doi.org/10.1007/s11154-009-9120-x

23 Gooley, J. J., Lu, J., Chou, T. C., Scammell, T. E., & Saper, C. B. (2001). Melanopsin in cells of origin of the retinohypothalamic tract. *Nature Neuroscience*, *4*(12), 1165–1165. https://doi.org/10.1038/nn768

24 Mohawk, J. A., Green, C. B., & Takahashi, J. S. (2012). Central and peripheral circadian clocks in mammals. *Annual Review of Neuroscience*, *35*, 445–462. https://doi.org/10.1146/annurev-neuro-060909-153128

25 Sasaki, H., Hattori, Y., Ikeda, Y., Kamagata, M., Iwami, S., Yasuda, S., & Shibata, S. (2016). Phase shifts in circadian peripheral clocks caused by exercise are dependent on the feeding schedule in PER2::LUC mice. *Chronobiology international*, *33*(7), 849–862. https://doi.org/10.3109/07420528.2016.1171775

26 Mistlberger, R. E. (2005). Circadian regulation of sleep in mammals: Role of the suprachiasmatic nucleus. *Brain Research Reviews, 49*(3), 429–454. https://doi.org/10.1016/j.brainresrev.2005.01.005

The Oldest Clock on Earth

27 Fang, M., LiWang, A., Golden, S. S., & Partch, C. L. (2024). The inner workings of an ancient biological clock. *Trends in biochemical sciences, 49*(3), 236–246. https://doi.org/10.1016/j.tibs.2023.12.007

28 Siebieszuk, A., Sejbuk, M., & Witkowska, A. M. (2023). Studying the human microbiota: Advances in understanding the fundamentals, origin, and evolution of biological timekeeping. *International Journal of Molecular Sciences, 24*(22), 16169. https://doi.org/10.3390/ijms242216169

29 Bell-Pedersen, D., Cassone, V. M., Earnest, D. J., Golden, S. S., Hardin, P. E., Thomas, T. L., & Zoran, M. J. (2005). Circadian rhythms from multiple oscillators: Lessons from diverse organisms. *Nature Reviews Genetics, 6*(7), 544–556. https://doi.org/10.1038/nrg1633

30 McClung C. R. (2006). Plant circadian rhythms. *The Plant cell, 18*(4), 792–803. https://doi.org/10.1105/tpc.106.040980

31 Fagiani, F., Di Marino, D., Romagnoli, A., Travelli, C., Voltan, D., Di Cesare Mannelli, L., Racchi, M., Govoni, S., & Lanni, C. (2022). Molecular regulations of circadian rhythm and implications for physiology and diseases. *Signal transduction and targeted therapy, 7*(1), 41. https://doi.org/10.1038/s41392-022-00899-y

32 Mihut, A., O'Neill, J. S., Partch, C. L., & Crosby, P. (2025). PERspectives on circadian cell biology. *Philosophical Transactions of the Royal Society B: Biological Sciences, 380*(1894), 20230483. https://doi.org/10.1098/rstb.2023.0483

33 Kuhlman, S. J., Craig, L. M., & Duffy, J. F. (2018). Introduction to Chronobiology. *Cold Spring Harbor perspectives in biology, 10*(9), a033613. https://doi.org/10.1101/cshperspect.a033613

34 Scott, H., Guyett, A., Manners, J., Stuart, N., Kemps, E., Toson, B., Lovato, N., Vakulin, A., Lack, L., & Banks, S. (2024). Circadian-informed lighting improves vigilance, sleep, and subjective sleepiness during simulated night-shift work. *Sleep, 47*(11), zsae173. https://doi.org/10.1093/sleep/zsae173

35 Crowley, S. J., Lee, C., Tseng, C. Y., Fogg, L. F., & Eastman, C. I. (2004). Complete or partial circadian re-entrainment improves performance, alertness, and mood during night-shift work. *Sleep*, *27*(6), 1077–1087. https://doi.org/10.1093/sleep/27.6.1077

The Hidden Metabolic Gatekeepers

36 Hariri, A., Mirian, M., Zarrabi, A., Kohandel, M., Amini-Pozveh, M., Aref, A. R., Tabatabaee, A., Prabhakar, P. K., & Sivakumar, P. M. (2023). The circadian rhythm: an influential soundtrack in the diabetes story. *Frontiers in endocrinology*, *14*, 1156757. https://doi.org/10.3389/fendo.2023.1156757

37 Morris, C. J., Purvis, T. E., Mistretta, J., Hu, K., & Scheer, F. A. J. L. (2017). Circadian Misalignment Increases C-Reactive Protein and Blood Pressure in Chronic Shift Workers. *Journal of biological rhythms*, *32*(2), 154–164. https://doi.org/10.1177/0748730417697537

38 Bautista, J., Ojeda-Mosquera, S., Ordóñez-Lozada, D., & López-Cortés, A. (2025). Peripheral clocks and systemic zeitgeber interactions: From molecular mechanisms to circadian precision medicine. *Frontiers in Endocrinology*, *16*, Article 1606242. https://doi.org/10.3389/fendo.2025.1606242

39 Duez, H., & Staels, B. (2025). Circadian Disruption and the Risk of Developing Obesity. *Current obesity reports*, *14*(1), 20. https://doi.org/10.1007/s13679-025-00610-6

40 Richard, A. J., White, U., Elks, C. M., et al. (2020, April 4). *Adipose tissue: Physiology to metabolic dysfunction*. In K. R. Feingold, S. F. Ahmed, B. Anawalt, et al. (Eds.), *Endotext*. MDText.com, Inc. https://www.ncbi.nlm.nih.gov/books/NBK555602/

41 Woller, A., & Gonze, D. (2021). Circadian Misalignment and Metabolic Disorders: A Story of Twisted Clocks. *Biology*, *10*(3), 207. https://doi.org/10.3390/biology10030207

42 Bescos, R., Boden, M. J., Jackson, M. L., Trewin, A. J., Marin, E. C., Levinger, I., Garnham, A., Hiam, D. S., Falcao-Tebas, F., Conte, F., Owens, J. A., Kennaway, D. J., & McConell, G. K. (2018). Four days of simulated shift work reduces insulin sensitivity in humans. *Acta physiologica (Oxford, England)*, *223*(2), e13039. https://doi.org/10.1111/apha.13039

43   Roenneberg, T., Winnebeck, E. C., & Klerman, E. B. (2019). Daylight
     Saving Time and Artificial Time Zones - A Battle Between Biological and
     Social Times. *Frontiers in physiology*, *10*, 944. https://doi.org/10.3389/
     fphys.2019.00944

44   Dyar, K. A., & Eckel-Mahan, K. L. (2017). Circadian Metabolomics
     in Time and Space. *Frontiers in neuroscience*, *11*, 369. https://doi.
     org/10.3389/fnins.2017.00369

45   Bass J. (2012). Circadian topology of metabolism. *Nature*, *491*(7424),
     348–356. https://doi.org/10.1038/nature11704

β-Cell Failure and the Rise of Diabetes

46   Halban, P. A., Polonsky, K. S., Bowden, D. W., Hawkins, M. A.,
     Ling, C., Mather, K. J., Powers, A. C., Rhodes, C. J., Sussel, L., &
     Weir, G. C. (2014). β-cell failure in type 2 diabetes: postulated
     mechanisms and prospects for prevention and treatment. *The Journal
     of clinical endocrinology and metabolism*, *99*(6), 1983–1992. https://doi.
     org/10.1210/jc.2014-1425

47   Gan, Y., Yang, C., Tong, X., Sun, H., Cong, Y., Yin, X., Li, L., Cao,
     S., Dong, X., Gong, Y., Shi, O., Deng, J., Bi, H., & Lu, Z. (2015).
     Shift work and diabetes mellitus: a meta-analysis of observational
     studies. *Occupational and environmental medicine*, *72*(1), 72–78.
     https://doi.org/10.1136/oemed-2014-102150

48   Buxton, O. M., Cain, S. W., O'Connor, S. P., Porter, J. H., Duffy, J.
     F., Wang, W., Czeisler, C. A., & Shea, S. A. (2012). Adverse metabolic
     consequences in humans of prolonged sleep restriction combined with
     circadian disruption. *Science translational medicine*, *4*(129), 129ra43.
     https://doi.org/10.1126/scitranslmed.3003200

49   Lee, J., Ma, K., Moulik, M., & Yechoor, V. (2018). Untimely oxidative
     stress in β-cells leads to diabetes – Role of circadian clock in β-cell
     function. *Free Radical Biology and Medicine*, *119*, 121–129. https://doi.
     org/10.1016/j.freeradbiomed.2018.02.022

50   Qian, J., Block, G. D., Colwell, C. S., & Matveyenko, A. V. (2013).
     Consequences of exposure to light at night on the pancreatic islet
     circadian clock and function in rats. *Diabetes*, *62*(10), 3469–3478.
     https://doi.org/10.2337/db12-1543

51 Haldar, S., Egli, L., De Castro, C. A., Tay, S. L., Koh, M. X. N., Darimont, C., Mace, K., & Henry, C. J. (2020). High or low glycemic index (GI) meals at dinner results in greater postprandial glycemia compared with breakfast: a randomized controlled trial. *BMJ open diabetes research & care*, *8*(1), e001099. https://doi.org/10.1136/bmjdrc-2019-001099

The Silenced Signal

52 Friedman J. M. (2011). Leptin and the regulation of body weigh. *The Keio journal of medicine*, *60*(1), 1–9. https://doi.org/10.2302/kjm.60.1

53 Obradovic, M., Sudar-Milovanovic, E., Soskic, S., Essack, M., Arya, S., Stewart, A. J., Gojobori, T., & Isenovic, E. R. (2021). Leptin and Obesity: Role and Clinical Implication. *Frontiers in endocrinology*, *12*, 585887. https://doi.org/10.3389/fendo.2021.585887

54 Spiegel, K., Leproult, R., & Van Cauter, E. (1999). Impact of sleep debt on metabolic and endocrine function. *Lancet (London, England)*, *354*(9188), 1435–1439. https://doi.org/10.1016/S0140-6736(99)01376-8

55 Otway, D. T., Mäntele, S., Bretschneider, S., Wright, J., Trayhurn, P., Skene, D. J., Robertson, M. D., & Johnston, J. D. (2011). Rhythmic diurnal gene expression in human adipose tissue from individuals who are lean, overweight, and type 2 diabetic. *Diabetes, 60*(5), 1577–1581. https://doi.org/10.2337/db10-1098

56 Wang, X., Takahashi, J. S., & Bass, J. (2010). Disruption of the clock components CLOCK and BMAL1 leads to hypoinsulinaemia and diabetes. *Nature, 466*(7306), 627–631. https://doi.org/10.1038/nature09253

57 Cedernaes, J., & Bass, J. (2021). You are when you eat: On circadian timing and energy balance. *Journal of Clinical Investigation, 131*(1), e144655. https://doi.org/10.1172/JCI144655

58 Myers, M. G., Cowley, M. A., & Münzberg, H. (2008). Mechanisms of leptin action and leptin resistance. *Annual review of physiology, 70*, 537–556. https://doi.org/10.1146/annurev.physiol.70.113006.100707

59 Taheri, S., Lin, L., Austin, D., Young, T., & Mignot, E. (2004). Short sleep duration is associated with reduced leptin, elevated ghrelin, and increased body mass index. *PLoS medicine*, *1*(3), e62. https://doi.org/10.1371/journal.pmed.0010062

60   Vilariño-García, T., Polonio-González, M. L., Pérez-Pérez, A., Ribalta, J., Arrieta, F., Aguilar, M., Obaya, J. C., Gimeno-Orna, J. A., Iglesias, P., Navarro, J., Durán, S., Pedro-Botet, J., & Sánchez-Margalet, V. (2024). Role of Leptin in Obesity, Cardiovascular Disease, and Type 2 Diabetes. *International journal of molecular sciences*, *25*(4), 2338. https://doi.org/10.3390/ijms25042338

61   Perakakis, N., & Mantzoros, C. S. (2024). Evidence from clinical studies of leptin: current and future clinical applications in humans. *Metabolism: clinical and experimental*, *161*, 156053. https://doi.org/10.1016/j. metabol.2024.156053

Microbial Rhythms and the Metabolic Toll

62   Alvarez, Y., Glotfelty, L. G., Blank, N., Dohnalová, L., & Thaiss, C. A. (2020). The Microbiome as a Circadian Coordinator of Metabolism. *Endocrinology*, *161*(6), bqaa059. https://doi.org/10.1210/ endocr/bqaa059

63   Thaiss, C. A., Zeevi, D., Levy, M., Zilberman-Schapira, G., Suez, J., Tengeler, A. C., Abramson, L., Katz, M. N., Korem, T., Zmora, N., Kuperman, Y., Biton, I., Gilad, S., Harmelin, A., Shapiro, H., Halpern, Z., Segal, E., & Elinav, E. (2014). Transkingdom control of microbiota diurnal oscillations promotes metabolic homeostasis. *Cell*, *159*(3), 514–529. https://doi.org/10.1016/j.cell.2014.09.048

64   Voigt, R. M., Forsyth, C. B., & Keshavarzian, A. (2019). Circadian rhythms: a regulator of gastrointestinal health and dysfunction. *Expert review of gastroenterology & hepatology*, *13*(5), 411–424. https://doi.org /10.1080/17474124.2019.1595588

65   Zarrinpar, A., Chaix, A., & Panda, S. (2016). Daily Eating Patterns and Their Impact on Health and Disease. *Trends in endocrinology and metabolism: TEM*, *27*(2), 69–83. https://doi.org/10.1016/j. tem.2015.11.007

66   Schrader, L. A., Ronnekleiv-Kelly, S. M., Hogenesch, J. B., Bradfield, C. A., & Malecki, K. M. (2024). Circadian disruption, clock genes, and metabolic health. *The Journal of clinical investigation*, *134*(14), e170998. https://doi.org/10.1172/JCI170998

67 Leone, V., Gibbons, S. M., Martinez, K., Hutchison, A. L., Huang, E. Y., Cham, C. M., Pierre, J. F., Heneghan, A. F., Nadimpalli, A., Hubert, N., Zale, E., Wang, Y., Huang, Y., Theriault, B., Dinner, A. R., Musch, M. W., Kudsk, K. A., Prendergast, B. J., Gilbert, J. A., & Chang, E. B. (2015). Effects of diurnal variation of gut microbes and high-fat feeding on host circadian clock function and metabolism. *Cell host & microbe*, *17*(5), 681–689. https://doi.org/10.1016/j.chom.2015.03.006

68 Spiegel, K., Tasali, E., Penev, P., & Van Cauter, E. (2004). Brief communication: Sleep curtailment in healthy young men is associated with decreased leptin levels, elevated ghrelin levels, and increased hunger and appetite. *Annals of internal medicine*, *141*(11), 846–850. https://doi.org/10.7326/0003-4819-141-11-200412070-00008

69 Leproult, R., & Van Cauter, E. (2010). Role of sleep and sleep loss in hormonal release and metabolism. *Endocrine development*, *17*, 11–21. https://doi.org/10.1159/000262524

70 Benedict, C., Vogel, H., Jonas, W., Woting, A., Blaut, M., Schürmann, A., & Cedernaes, J. (2016). Gut microbiota and glucometabolic alterations in response to recurrent partial sleep deprivation in normal-weight young individuals. *Molecular metabolism*, *5*(12), 1175–1186. https://doi.org/10.1016/j.molmet.2016.10.003

71 Bishehsari, F., Voigt, R. M., & Keshavarzian, A. (2020). Circadian rhythms and the gut microbiota: from the metabolic syndrome to cancer. *Nature reviews. Endocrinology*, *16*(12), 731–739. https://doi.org/10.1038/s41574-020-00427-4

72 Gibson, G. R., Hutkins, R., Sanders, M. E., Prescott, S. L., Reimer, R. A., Salminen, S. J., Scott, K., Stanton, C., Swanson, K. S., Cani, P. D., Verbeke, K., & Reid, G. (2017). The International Scientific Association for Probiotics and Prebiotics (ISAPP) consensus statement on the definition and scope of prebiotics. *Nature Reviews Gastroenterology & Hepatology*, *14*(8), 491–502. https://doi.org/10.1038/nrgastro.2017.75

Interlude: What Aristotle Knew That Shift Workers Forget

73 Bernacer, J., & Murillo, J. I. (2014). The Aristotelian conception of habit and its contribution to human neuroscience. *Frontiers in human neuroscience*, *8*, 883. https://doi.org/10.3389/fnhum.2014.00883

Shift Work and Female Rhythm Disruption

74   Baker, F. C., & Lee, K. A. (2022). Menstrual Cycle Effects on Sleep. *Sleep medicine clinics*, *17*(2), 283–294. https://doi.org/10.1016/j.jsmc.2022.02.004

75   Lawson, C. C., Johnson, C. Y., Chavarro, J. E., Lividoti Hibert, E. N., Whelan, E. A., Rocheleau, C. M., Grajewski, B., Schernhammer, E. S., & Rich-Edwards, J. W. (2015). Work schedule and physically demanding work in relation to menstrual function: the Nurses' Health Study 3. Scandinavian journal of work, environment & health, 41(2), 194–203. https://doi.org/10.5271/sjweh.3482

76   Shechter, A., & Boivin, D. B. (2010). Sleep, Hormones, and Circadian Rhythms throughout the Menstrual Cycle in Healthy Women and Women with Premenstrual Dysphoric Disorder. *International journal of endocrinology*, *2010*, 259345. https://doi.org/10.1155/2010/259345

77   Baker, F. C., Waner, J. I., Vieira, E. F., Taylor, S. R., Driver, H. S., & Mitchell, D. (2001). Sleep and 24 hour body temperatures: a comparison in young men, naturally cycling women and women taking hormonal contraceptives. *The Journal of physiology*, *530*(Pt 3), 565–574. https://doi.org/10.1111/j.1469-7793.2001.0565k.x

78   Karman, B. N., & Tischkau, S. A. (2006). Circadian clock gene expression in the ovary: Effects of luteinizing hormone. *Biology of reproduction*, *75*(4), 624–632. https://doi.org/10.1095/biolreprod.106.050732

79   Olcese J. M. (2020). Melatonin and Female Reproduction: An Expanding Universe. *Frontiers in endocrinology*, *11*, 85. https://doi.org/10.3389/fendo.2020.00085

80   Basini, G., & Grasselli, F. (2024). Role of Melatonin in Ovarian Function. *Animals : an open access journal from MDPI*, *14*(4), 644. https://doi.org/10.3390/ani14040644

81   Marseglia, L., Gitto, E., Laschi, E., Giordano, M., Romeo, C., Cannavò, L., Toni, A. L., Buonocore, G., & Perrone, S. (2021). Antioxidant Effect of Melatonin in Preterm Newborns. Oxidative medicine and cellular longevity, 2021, 6308255. https://doi.org/10.1155/2021/6308255

82 Stock, D., Knight, J. A., Raboud, J., Cotterchio, M., Strohmaier, S., Willett, W., Eliassen, A. H., Rosner, B., Hankinson, S. E., & Schernhammer, E. (2019). Rotating night shift work and menopausal age. *Human reproduction (Oxford, England)*, *34*(3), 539–548. https://doi.org/10.1093/humrep/dey390

83 Hu, F., Wu, C., Jia, Y., Zhen, H., Cheng, H., Zhang, F., Wang, L., & Jiang, M. (2023). Shift work and menstruation: A meta-analysis study. *SSM - population health*, *24*, 101542. https://doi.org/10.1016/j.ssmph.2023.101542

84 Zhu, J. L., Hjollund, N. H., Andersen, A. M., & Olsen, J. (2004). Shift work, job stress, and late fetal loss: The National Birth Cohort in Denmark. *Journal of occupational and environmental medicine*, *46*(11), 1144–1149. https://doi.org/10.1097/01.jom.0000145168.21614.21

85 Silva, I., & Costa, D. (2023). Consequences of Shift Work and Night Work: A Literature Review. *Healthcare (Basel, Switzerland)*, *11*(10), 1410. https://doi.org/10.3390/healthcare11101410

86 Ryczkowska, K., Adach, W., Janikowski, K., Banach, M., & Bielecka-Dabrowa, A. (2022). Menopause and women's cardiovascular health: is it really an obvious relationship?. *Archives of medical science : AMS*, *19*(2), 458–466. https://doi.org/10.5114/aoms/157308

How Shift Work Breaks Male Hormonal Rhythms

87 Brambilla, D. J., Matsumoto, A. M., Araujo, A. B., & McKinlay, J. B. (2009). The effect of diurnal variation on clinical measurement of serum testosterone and other sex hormone levels in men. *The Journal of clinical endocrinology and metabolism*, *94*(3), 907–913. https://doi.org/10.1210/jc.2008-1902

88 Liu, P. Y., Beilin, J., Meier, C., Nguyen, T. V., Center, J. R., Leedman, P. J., Seibel, M. J., Eisman, J. A., & Handelsman, D. J. (2007). Age-related changes in serum testosterone and sex hormone binding globulin in Australian men: longitudinal analyses of two geographically separate regional cohorts. *The Journal of clinical endocrinology and metabolism*, *92*(9), 3599–3603. https://doi.org/10.1210/jc.2007-0862

89 Scheer, F. A., Hilton, M. F., Mantzoros, C. S., & Shea, S. A. (2009). Adverse metabolic and cardiovascular consequences of circadian misalignment. *Proceedings of the National Academy of Sciences of the United States of America, 106*(11), 4453–4458. https://doi.org/10.1073/pnas.0808180106

90 Zheng, Z., Pan, J., Chen, Z., Gao, P., Gao, J., Jiang, H., & Zhang, X. (2024). The association between shift work, shift work sleep disorders and premature ejaculation in male workers. *BMC public health, 24*(1), 1772. https://doi.org/10.1186/s12889-024-19141-1

91 Durmer, J. S., & Dinges, D. F. (2005). Neurocognitive consequences of sleep deprivation. *Seminars in neurology, 25*(1), 117–129. https://doi.org/10.1055/s-2005-867080

92 Andersen, M. L., Alvarenga, T. F., Mazaro-Costa, R., Hachul, H. C., & Tufik, S. (2011). The association of testosterone, sleep, and sexual function in men and women. *Brain research, 1416*, 80–104. https://doi.org/10.1016/j.brainres.2011.07.060

93 Demirkol, M. K., Yıldırım, A., Gıca, Ş., Doğan, N. T., & Resim, S. (2021). Evaluation of the effect of shift working and sleep quality on semen parameters in men attending infertility clinic. *Andrologia, 53*(8), e14116. https://doi.org/10.1111/and.14116

94 Chen, H.-G., Sun, B., Chen, Y.-J., Chavarro, J. E., Hu, S.-H., Xiong, C.-L., Pan, A., Meng, T.-Q., Wang, Y.-X., & Messerlian, C. (2020). Sleep duration and quality in relation to semen quality in healthy men screened as potential sperm donors. *Environment International, 134*, 105368. https://doi.org/10.1016/j.envint.2019.105368

Compromised Vascular Infrastructure

95 Vetter, C., Devore, E. E., Wegrzyn, L. R., Massa, J., Speizer, F. E., Kawachi, I., Rosner, B., Stampfer, M. J., & Schernhammer, E. S. (2016). Association Between Rotating Night Shift Work and Risk of Coronary Heart Disease Among Women. *JAMA, 315*(16), 1726–1734. https://doi.org/10.1001/jama.2016.4454

96 Torquati, L., Mielke, G. I., Brown, W. J., & Kolbe-Alexander, T. (2018). Shift work and the risk of cardiovascular disease. A systematic review and meta-analysis including dose-response relationship. *Scandinavian journal of work, environment & health, 44*(3), 229–238. https://doi.org/10.5271/sjweh.3700

97 Bermudez, E. A., Rifai, N., Buring, J., Manson, J. E., & Ridker, P. M. (2002). Interrelationships among circulating interleukin-6, C-reactive protein, and traditional cardiovascular risk factors in women. *Arteriosclerosis, thrombosis, and vascular biology*, *22*(10), 1668–1673. https://doi.org/10.1161/01.atv.0000029781.31325.66

98 Libby P. (2021). The changing landscape of athero-sclerosis. *Nature*, *592*(7855), 524–533. https://doi.org/10.1038/s41586-021-03392-8

99 Anea, C. B., Zhang, M., Stepp, D. W., Simkins, G. B., Reed, G., Fulton, D. J., & Rudic, R. D. (2009). Vascular disease in mice with a dysfunctional circadian clock. *Circulation*, *119*(11), 1510–1517. https://doi.org/10.1161/CIRCULATIONAHA.108.827477

100 Thosar, S. S., Berman, A. M., Herzig, M. X., McHill, A. W., Bowles, N. P., Swanson, C. M., Clemons, N. A., Butler, M. P., Clemons, A. A., Emens, J. S., & Shea, S. A. (2019). Circadian Rhythm of Vascular Function in Midlife Adults. *Arteriosclerosis, thrombosis, and vascular biology*, *39*(6), 1203–1211. https://doi.org/10.1161/ATVBAHA.119.312682

101 Dutheil, F., Fournier, A., Perrier, C., Richard, D., Trousselard, M., Mnatzaganian, G., Baker, J. S., Bagheri, R., Mermillod, M., Clinchamps, M., Schmidt, J., & Bouillon-Minois, J. B. (2024). Impact of 24 h shifts on urinary catecholamine in emergency physicians: a cross-over randomized trial. *Scientific reports*, *14*(1), 7329. https://doi.org/10.1038/s41598-024-58070-2

102 Grassi G. (2006). Sympathetic overdrive and cardiovascular risk in the metabolic syndrome. *Hypertension research : official journal of the Japanese Society of Hypertension*, *29*(11), 839–847. https://doi.org/10.1291/hypres.29.839

When the Heart Falls Out Of Time

103 Chan, B., Buckley, T., Hansen, P., Shaw, E., & Tofler, G. H. (2023). Circadian variation in acute myocardial infarction and modification by coronary artery disease: a prospective observational study. *European heart journal open*, *3*(4), oead068. https://doi.org/10.1093/ehjopen/oead068

104   Fodor, D. M., Marta, M. M., & Perju-Dumbravă, L. (2021). Implications of Circadian Rhythm in Stroke Occurrence: Certainties and Possibilities. *Brain sciences, 11*(7), 865. https://doi.org/10.3390/brainsci11070865

105   Scheer, F. A., Hu, K., Evoniuk, H., Kelly, E. E., Malhotra, A., Hilton, M. F., & Shea, S. A. (2010). Impact of the human circadian system, exercise, and their interaction on cardiovascular function. *Proceedings of the National Academy of Sciences of the United States of America, 107*(47), 20541–20546. https://doi.org/10.1073/pnas.1006749107

106   Puttonen, S., Härmä, M., & Hublin, C. (2010). Shift work and cardiovascular disease - pathways from circadian stress to morbidity. *Scandinavian journal of work, environment & health, 36*(2), 96–108. https://doi.org/10.5271/sjweh.2894

107   Ashor, A. W., Lara, J., Siervo, M., Celis-Morales, C., & Mathers, J. C. (2014). Effects of exercise modalities on arterial stiffness and wave reflection: A systematic review and meta-analysis of randomized controlled trials. *PLOS ONE, 9*(10), e110034. https://doi.org/10.1371/journal.pone.0110034

108   Lavie, C. J., Arena, R., Swift, D. L., Johannsen, N. M., Sui, X., Lee, D. C., Earnest, C. P., Church, T. S., O'Keefe, J. H., Milani, R. V., & Blair, S. N. (2015). Exercise and the cardiovascular system: clinical science and cardiovascular outcomes. *Circulation research, 117*(2), 207–219. https://doi.org/10.1161/CIRCRESAHA.117.305205

109   Weston, K. S., Wisløff, U., & Coombes, J. S. (2014). High-intensity interval training in patients with lifestyle-induced cardiometabolic disease: a systematic review and meta-analysis. *British journal of sports medicine, 48*(16), 1227–1234. https://doi.org/10.1136/bjsports-2013-092576

How Fat Turns Against Us

110   Fasshauer, M., & Blüher, M. (2015). Adipokines in health and disease. *Trends in pharmacological sciences, 36*(7), 461–470. https://doi.org/10.1016/j.tips.2015.04.014

111   Kettner, N. M., Mayo, S. A., Hua, J., Lee, C., Moore, D. D., & Fu, L. (2015). Circadian Dysfunction Induces Leptin Resistance in Mice. *Cell metabolism, 22*(3), 448–459. https://doi.org/10.1016/j.cmet.2015.06.005

112   McNeill, B. T., Suchacki, K. J., & Stimson, R. H. (2021). MECHANISMS IN ENDOCRINOLOGY: Human brown adipose tissue as a therapeutic target: warming up or cooling down?. *European journal of endocrinology, 184*(6), R243–R259. https://doi.org/10.1530/EJE-20-1439

113   Greco, C. M., & Sassone-Corsi, P. (2019). Circadian blueprint of metabolic pathways in the brain. *Nature reviews. Neuroscience, 20*(2), 71–82. https://doi.org/10.1038/s41583-018-0096-y

114   Xie, Z., Tang, Y., & Wang, Y. (2021). Circadian rhythms and obesity: Timekeeping governs lipid metabolism. *Chronic Diseases and Translational Medicine, 7*(1), 13–21. https://doi.org/10.1097/CM9.0000000000000702

115   Leinweber, B., Pilorz, V., Olejniczak, I., Skrum, L., Begemann, K., Heyde, I., Stenger, S., Sadik, C. D., & Oster, H. (2025). *Bmal1* deficiency in neutrophils alleviates symptoms induced by high-fat diet. *iScience, 28*(3), 112038. https://doi.org/10.1016/j.isci.2025.112038

116   Yue, K., Rensen, P. C. N., & Kooijman, S. (2023). Circadian control of white and brown adipose tissues. *Current Opinion in Genetics & Development, 81*, 102056. https://doi.org/10.1016/j.gde.2023.102056

117   Chan, K., Wong, F. S., & Pearson, J. A. (2022). Circadian rhythms and pancreas physiology: A review. *Frontiers in endocrinology, 13*, 920261. https://doi.org/10.3389/fendo.2022.920261

118   Regmi, P., & Heilbronn, L. K. (2020). Time-Restricted Eating: Benefits, Mechanisms, and Challenges in Translation. *iScience, 23*(6), 101161. https://doi.org/10.1016/j.isci.2020.101161

119   Froy, O., & Garaulet, M. (2018). The Circadian Clock in White and Brown Adipose Tissue: Mechanistic, Endocrine, and Clinical Aspects. *Endocrine reviews, 39*(3), 261–273. https://doi.org/10.1210/er.2017-00193

The Silent Organ Shift

120   Mukherji, A., Bailey, S. M., Staels, B., & Baumert, T. F. (2019). The circadian clock and liver function in health and disease. *Journal of hepatology, 71*(1), 200–211. https://doi.org/10.1016/j.jhep.2019.03.020

121 Wang, F., Zhang, L., Wu, S., Li, W., Sun, M., Feng, W., Ding, D., Yeung-Shan Wong, S., Zhu, P., Evans, G. J., Wing, Y. K., Zhang, J., Vlaanderen, J. J., Vermeulen, R. C. H., Zhang, Y., Chan, E. Y., Li, Z., & Tse, L. A. (2019). Night shift work and abnormal liver function: is non-alcohol fatty liver a necessary mediator?. *Occupational and environmental medicine*, *76*(2), 83–89. https://doi.org/10.1136/oemed-2018-105273

122 Sharma, B., & John, S. (2023, April 7). Nonalcoholic steatohepatitis (NASH). In *StatPearls*. StatPearls Publishing. https://www.ncbi.nlm.nih.gov/books/NBK470243/

123 Sun, J., Mao, S., & Lu, C. (2025). Association between circadian syndrome and MASLD risk: evidence from a large cross-sectional study. *BMC gastroenterology*, *25*(1), 391. https://doi.org/10.1186/s12876-025-03997-7

124 Wefers, J., van Moorsel, D., Hansen, J., Connell, N. J., Havekes, B., Hoeks, J., van Marken Lichtenbelt, W. D., Duez, H., Phielix, E., Kalsbeek, A., Boekschoten, M. V., Hooiveld, G. J., Hesselink, M. K. C., Kersten, S., Staels, B., Scheer, F. A. J. L., & Schrauwen, P. (2018). Circadian misalignment induces fatty acid metabolism gene profiles and compromises insulin sensitivity in human skeletal muscle. *Proceedings of the National Academy of Sciences of the United States of America*, *115*(30), 7789–7794. https://doi.org/10.1073/pnas.1722295115

125 Hariri, A., Mirian, M., Zarrabi, A., Kohandel, M., Amini-Pozveh, M., Aref, A. R., Tabatabaee, A., Prabhakar, P. K., & Sivakumar, P. M. (2023). The circadian rhythm: An influential soundtrack in the diabetes story. *Frontiers in Endocrinology*, *14*, Article 1156757. https://doi.org/10.3389/fendo.2023.1156757

126 Tran, H. T., Kondo, T., Ashry, A., Fu, Y., Okawa, H., Sawangmake, C., & Egusa, H. (2024). Effect of circadian clock disruption on type 2 diabetes. *Frontiers in physiology*, *15*, 1435848. https://doi.org/10.3389/fphys.2024.1435848

127 Gilani, A., Pandey, V., Garcia, V., Agostinucci, K., Singh, S. P., Schragenheim, J., Bellner, L., Falck, J. R., Paudyal, M. P., Capdevila, J. H., Abraham, N. G., & Laniado Schwartzman, M. (2018). High-fat diet-induced obesity and insulin resistance in CYP4a14$^{-/-}$ mice is mediated by 20-HETE. *American journal of physiology. Regulatory, integrative and comparative physiology*, *315*(5), R934–R944. https://doi.org/10.1152/ajpregu.00125.2018

128   Sadacca, L. A., Lamia, K. A., deLemos, A. S., Blum, B., & Weitz, C. J. (2011). An intrinsic circadian clock of the pancreas is required for normal insulin release and glucose homeostasis in mice. *Diabetologia*, *54*(1), 120–124. https://doi.org/10.1007/s00125-010-1920-8

How Circadian Rhythms Shape Strength

129   Wolff, G., & Esser, K. A. (2012). Scheduled exercise phase shifts the circadian clock in skeletal muscle. *Medicine and science in sports and exercise*, *44*(9), 1663–1670. https://doi.org/10.1249/MSS.0b013e318255cf4c

130   Viggars, M. R., Berko, H. E., Hesketh, S. J., Wolff, C. A., Gutierrez-Monreal, M. A., Martin, R. A., Jennings, I. G., Huo, Z., & Esser, K. A. (2024). Skeletal muscle BMAL1 is necessary for transcriptional adaptation of local and peripheral tissues in response to endurance exercise training. *Molecular metabolism*, *86*, 101980. https://doi.org/10.1016/j.molmet.2024.101980

131   Andrews, J. L., Zhang, X., McCarthy, J. J., McDearmon, E. L., Hornberger, T. A., Russell, B., Campbell, K. S., Arbogast, S., Reid, M. B., Walker, J. R., Hogenesch, J. B., Takahashi, J. S., & Esser, K. A. (2010). CLOCK and BMAL1 regulate MyoD and are necessary for maintenance of skeletal muscle phenotype and function. *Proceedings of the National Academy of Sciences of the United States of America*, *107*(44), 19090–19095. https://doi.org/10.1073/pnas.1014523107

Top of Form

132   Lamon, S., Morabito, A., Arentson-Lantz, E., Knowles, O., Vincent, G. E., Condo, D., Alexander, S. E., Garnham, A., Paddon-Jones, D., & Aisbett, B. (2021). The effect of acute sleep deprivation on skeletal muscle protein synthesis and the hormonal environment. *Physiological reports*, *9*(1), e14660. https://doi.org/10.14814/phy2.14660

133   Nedeltcheva, A. V., Kilkus, J. M., Imperial, J., Kasza, K., Schoeller, D. A., & Penev, P. D. (2009). Sleep curtailment is accompanied by increased intake of calories from snacks. *The American journal of clinical nutrition*, *89*(1), 126–133. https://doi.org/10.3945/ajcn.2008.26574

134 Spiegel, K., Tasali, E., Penev, P., & Van Cauter, E. (2004). Brief communication: Sleep curtailment in healthy young men is associated with decreased leptin levels, elevated ghrelin levels, and increased hunger and appetite. *Annals of internal medicine, 141*(11), 846–850. https://doi.org/10.7326/0003-4819-141-11-200412070-00008

135 Phillips, S. M., & Van Loon, L. J. (2011). Dietary protein for athletes: from requirements to optimum adaptation. *Journal of sports sciences, 29 Suppl 1*, S29–S38. https://doi.org/10.1080/02640414.2011.619204

136 Schoenfeld, B. J., & Aragon, A. A. (2018). How much protein can the body use in a single meal for muscle-building? Implications for daily protein distribution. *Journal of the International Society of Sports Nutrition, 15*, 10. https://doi.org/10.1186/s12970-018-0215-1

137 Moore, D. R., Churchward-Venne, T. A., Witard, O., Breen, L., Burd, N. A., Tipton, K. D., & Phillips, S. M. (2015). Protein ingestion to stimulate myofibrillar protein synthesis requires greater relative protein intakes in healthy older versus younger men. *The journals of gerontology. Series A, Biological sciences and medical sciences, 70*(1), 57–62. https://doi.org/10.1093/gerona/glu103

138 Holten, M. K., Zacho, M., Gaster, M., Juel, C., Wojtaszewski, J. F., & Dela, F. (2004). Strength training increases insulin-mediated glucose uptake, GLUT4 content, and insulin signaling in skeletal muscle in patients with type 2 diabetes. *Diabetes, 53*(2), 294–305. https://doi.org/10.2337/diabetes.53.2.294

139 Feltz, D. L., Kerr, N. L., & Irwin, B. C. (2011). Buddy up: the Köhler effect applied to health games. *Journal of sport & exercise psychology, 33*(4), 506–526. https://doi.org/10.1123/jsep.33.4.506

The Fast-Forward Button on the Brain

140 Duhart, J. M., Inami, S., & Koh, K. (2023). Many faces of sleep regulation: beyond the time of day and prior wake time. *The FEBS journal, 290*(4), 931–950. https://doi.org/10.1111/febs.16320

141 Logan, R. W., & McClung, C. A. (2019). Rhythms of life: circadian disruption and brain disorders across the lifespan. *Nature reviews. Neuroscience, 20*(1), 49–65. https://doi.org/10.1038/s41583-018-0088-y

142 Li, X., He, Y., Wang, D., & Momeni, M. R. (2024). Chronobiological disruptions: unravelling the interplay of shift work, circadian rhythms, and vascular health in the context of stroke risk. *Clinical and experimental medicine*, *25*(1), 6. https://doi.org/10.1007/s10238-024-01514-w

143 Yook, S., Choi, S. J., Lee, H., Joo, E. Y., & Kim, H. (2024). Long-term night-shift work is associated with accelerates brain aging and worsens N3 sleep in female nurses. *Sleep medicine*, *121*, 69–76. https://doi.org/10.1016/j.sleep.2024.06.013

144 Park, S., Hong, H., Kim, R. Y., Ma, J., Lee, S., Ha, E., Yoon, S., & Kim, J. (2021). Firefighters Have Cerebral Blood Flow Reductions in the Orbitofrontal and Insular Cortices That are Associated with Poor Sleep Quality. *Nature and science of sleep*, *13*, 1507–1517. https://doi.org/10.2147/NSS.S312671

145 Cheng, P., Tallent, G., Anderson, C., Albrecht, M. A., & Drake, C. L. (2017). Shift work and cognitive flexibility: Decomposing task performance. *Journal of Biological Rhythms, 32*(2), 143–153. https://doi.org/10.1177/0748730417699309

146 Colten, H. R., & Altevogt, B. M. (Eds.). (2006). *Sleep disorders and sleep deprivation: An unmet public health problem* (Institute of Medicine (US) Committee on Sleep Medicine and Research). National Academies Press. https://www.ncbi.nlm.nih.gov/books/NBK19961/

Cancer and the Clock

147 Masri, S., & Sassone-Corsi, P. (2018). The emerging link between cancer, metabolism, and circadian rhythms. *Nature medicine*, *24*(12), 1795–1803. https://doi.org/10.1038/s41591-018-0271-8

148 Buhr, E. D., & Takahashi, J. S. (2013). Molecular components of the Mammalian circadian clock. *Handbook of experimental pharmacology*, (217), 3–27. https://doi.org/10.1007/978-3-642-25950-0_1

149 El-Tanani, M., Rabbani, S. A., Ali, A. A., Alfaouri, I. G. A., Al Nsairat, H., Al-Ani, I. H., Aljabali, A. A., Rizzo, M., Patoulias, D., Khan, M. A., Parvez, S., & El-Tanani, Y. (2024). Circadian rhythms and cancer: implications for timing in therapy. *Discover oncology*, *15*(1), 767. https://doi.org/10.1007/s12672-024-01643-4

150 Lee Y. (2021). Roles of circadian clocks in cancer pathogenesis and treatment. *Experimental & molecular medicine*, *53*(10), 1529–1538. https://doi.org/10.1038/s12276-021-00681-0

151 Sulli, G., Lam, M. T. Y., & Panda, S. (2019). Interplay between Circadian Clock and Cancer: New Frontiers for Cancer Treatment. *Trends in cancer*, *5*(8), 475–494. https://doi.org/10.1016/j.trecan.2019.07.002

152 Amjad, M. T., Chidharla, A., & Kasi, A. (2023, February 27). *Cancer chemotherapy*. In StatPearls. StatPearls Publishing. https://www.ncbi.nlm.nih.gov/books/NBK564367/

153 Dean, L., & Kane, M. (2016, November 3). *Fluorouracil therapy and DPYD genotype* (Updated 2021, January 11). In V. M. Pratt, S. A. Scott, M. Pirmohamed, et al. (Eds.), *Medical genetics summaries*. National Center for Biotechnology Information (US). https://www.ncbi.nlm.nih.gov/books/NBK395610/

154 Das, N. K., & Samanta, S. (2022). The potential anti-cancer effects of melatonin on breast cancer. *Exploration of Medicine*, *3*, 112–127. https://doi.org/10.37349/emed.2022.00078

155 Bautista, J., Ojeda-Mosquera, S., Ordóñez-Lozada, D., & López-Cortés, A. (2025). Peripheral clocks and systemic *zeitgeber* interactions: from molecular mechanisms to circadian precision medicine. *Frontiers in endocrinology*, *16*, 1606242. https://doi.org/10.3389/fendo.2025.1606242

156 Sulli, G., Lam, M. T. Y., & Panda, S. (2019). Interplay between Circadian Clock and Cancer: New Frontiers for Cancer Treatment. *Trends in cancer*, *5*(8), 475–494. https://doi.org/10.1016/j.trecan.2019.07.002

157 Zeng, Y., Guo, Z., Wu, M., Chen, F., & Chen, L. (2024). Circadian rhythm regulates the function of immune cells and participates in the development of tumors. *Cell Death Discovery*, *10*, Article 199. https://doi.org/10.1038/s41420-024-01734-6

Circadian Science in Critical Illness

158 Boots, R., Mead, G., Rawashdeh, O., Bellapart, J., Townsend, S., Paratz, J., Garner, N., Clement, P., Oddy, D., & Circadian Investigators in Critical Illness (2023). Circadian Hygiene in the ICU Environment (CHIE) study. *Critical care and resuscitation : journal of the Australasian Academy of Critical Care Medicine*, *22*(4), 361–369. https://doi.org/10.51893/2020.4.OA9

159   Sakr, Y., Jaschinski, U., Wittebole, X., Szakmany, T., Lipman, J., Ñamendys-Silva, S. A., Martin-Loeches, I., Leone, M., Lupu, M. N., Vincent, J. L., & ICON Investigators (2018). Sepsis in Intensive Care Unit Patients: Worldwide Data From the Intensive Care over Nations Audit. *Open forum infectious diseases*, 5(12), ofy313. https://doi.org/10.1093/ofid/ofy313

160   Ali, M., & Cascella, M. (2024, March 13). *ICU delirium*. In StatPearls. StatPearls Publishing. https://www.ncbi.nlm.nih.gov/books/NBK559280/

161   Nishikimi, M., Numaguchi, A., Takahashi, K., Miyagawa, Y., Matsui, K., Higashi, M., Makishi, G., Matsui, S., & Matsuda, N. (2018). Effect of Administration of Ramelteon, a Melatonin Receptor Agonist, on the Duration of Stay in the ICU: A Single-Center Randomized Placebo-Controlled Trial. *Critical care medicine*, 46(7), 1099–1105. https://doi.org/10.1097/CCM.0000000000003132

162   Prin, M., Bertazzo, J., Walker, L. A., Scott, B., & Eckle, T. (2023). Enhancing circadian rhythms-the circadian MEGA bundle as novel approach to treat critical illness. *Annals of translational medicine*, 11(9), 319. https://doi.org/10.21037/atm-22-5127

The Power Laws: Building Rhythm From What you Can Control

163   Nollet, M., Franks, N. P., & Wisden, W. (2023). Understanding Sleep Regulation in Normal and Pathological Conditions, and Why It Matters. *Journal of Huntington's disease*, 12(2), 105–119. https://doi.org/10.3233/JHD-230564

164   Mesarwi, O., Polak, J., Jun, J., & Polotsky, V. Y. (2013). Sleep disorders and the development of insulin resistance and obesity. *Endocrinology and metabolism clinics of North America*, 42(3), 617–634. https://doi.org/10.1016/j.ecl.2013.05.001

165   Hossain, M. N., Lee, J., Choi, H., Kwak, Y. S., & Kim, J. (2024). The impact of exercise on depression: how moving makes your brain and body feel better. *Physical activity and nutrition*, 28(2), 43–51. https://doi.org/10.20463/pan.2024.0015

166   Easton, D. F., Gupta, C. C., Vincent, G. E., & Ferguson, S. A. (2024). Move the night way: how can physical activity facilitate adaptation to shift work?. *Communications biology*, 7(1), 259. https://doi.org/10.1038/s42003-024-05962-8

When Sleep Fails, Everything Follows

167 National Institute of Neurological Disorders and Stroke. (2025). *Brain basics: Understanding sleep.* National Institutes of Health. https://www.ninds.nih.gov/health-information/public-education/brain-basics/brain-basics-understanding-sleep

168 Phillips, A. J. K., Klerman, E. B., & Butler, J. P. (2017). Modeling the adenosine system as a modulator of cognitive performance and sleep patterns during sleep restriction and recovery. *PLoS computational biology*, *13*(10), e1005759. https://doi.org/10.1371/journal.pcbi.1005759

169 Meléndez-Fernández, O. H., Liu, J. A., & Nelson, R. J. (2023). Circadian Rhythms Disrupted by Light at Night and Mistimed Food Intake Alter Hormonal Rhythms and Metabolism. *International journal of molecular sciences*, *24*(4), 3392. https://doi.org/10.3390/ijms24043392

170 Gandhi, A. V., Mosser, E. A., Oikonomou, G., & Prober, D. A. (2015). Melatonin is required for the circadian regulation of sleep. *Neuron*, *85*(6), 1193–1199. https://doi.org/10.1016/j.neuron.2015.02.016

171 Savarese, M., & Di Perri, M. C. (2020). Excessive sleepiness in shift work disorder: a narrative review of the last 5 years. *Sleep & breathing = Schlaf & Atmung*, *24*(1), 297–310. https://doi.org/10.1007/s11325-019-01925-0

172 Flo, E., Pallesen, S., Magerøy, N., Moen, B. E., Grønli, J., Nordhus, I. H., & Bjorvatn, B. (2012). Shift work disorder in nurses – Assessment, prevalence and related health problems. *PLOS ONE*, *7*(4), e33981. https://doi.org/10.1371/journal.pone.0033981

173 Membrive-Jiménez, M. J., Gómez-Urquiza, J. L., Suleiman-Martos, N., Velando-Soriano, A., Ariza, T., De la Fuente-Solana, E. I., & Cañadas-De la Fuente, G. A. (2022). Relation between Burnout and Sleep Problems in Nurses: A Systematic Review with Meta-Analysis. *Healthcare (Basel, Switzerland)*, *10*(5), 954. https://doi.org/10.3390/healthcare10050954

174 Ashbrook, L. H., Krystal, A. D., Fu, Y. H., & Ptáček, L. J. (2020). Genetics of the human circadian clock and sleep homeostat. *Neuropsychopharmacology : official publication of the American College of Neuropsychopharmacology*, *45*(1), 45–54. https://doi.org/10.1038/s41386-019-0476-7

175 Chaput, J. P., McHill, A. W., Cox, R. C., Broussard, J. L., Dutil, C., da Costa, B. G. G., Sampasa-Kanyinga, H., & Wright, K. P., Jr (2023). The role of insufficient sleep and circadian misalignment in obesity. *Nature reviews. Endocrinology, 19*(2), 82–97. https://doi.org/10.1038/s41574-022-00747-7

176 Goel, N., Rao, H., Durmer, J. S., & Dinges, D. F. (2009). Neurocognitive consequences of sleep deprivation. *Seminars in neurology, 29*(4), 320–339. https://doi.org/10.1055/s-0029-1237117

177 Ohara, M., & Hattori, T. (2025). The Glymphatic System in Cerebrospinal Fluid Dynamics: Clinical Implications, Its Evaluation, and Application to Therapeutics. *Neuro-degenerative diseases*, 1–13. Advance online publication. https://doi.org/10.1159/000546286

178 Shokri-Kojori, E., Wang, G., Wiers, C. E., Demiral, S. B., Guo, M., Kim, S. W., Lindgren, E., Ramirez, V., Zehra, A., Freeman, C., Miller, G., Manza, P., Srivastava, T., De Santi, S., Tomasi, D., Benveniste, H., & Volkow, N. D. (2018). β-Amyloid accumulation in the human brain after one night of sleep deprivation. *Proceedings of the National Academy of Sciences of the United States of America, 115*(17), 4483–4488. https://doi.org/10.1073/pnas.1721694115

179 National Institutes of Health. (2019, September 24). *Gene identified in people who need little sleep*. NIH Research Matters. https://www.nih.gov/news-events/nih-research-matters/gene-identified-people-who-need-little-sleep

180 Emens, J. S., & Burgess, H. J. (2015). Effect of Light and Melatonin and Other Melatonin Receptor Agonists on Human Circadian Physiology. *Sleep medicine clinics, 10*(4), 435–453. https://doi.org/10.1016/j.jsmc.2015.08.001

Nutrition as a Strategy for Survival

181 Dakanalis, A., Mentzelou, M., Papadopoulou, S. K., Papandreou, D., Spanoudaki, M., Vasios, G. K., Pavlidou, E., Mantzorou, M., & Giaginis, C. (2023). The Association of Emotional Eating with Overweight/Obesity, Depression, Anxiety/Stress, and Dietary Patterns: A Review of the Current Clinical Evidence. *Nutrients, 15*(5), 1173. https://doi.org/10.3390/nu15051173

182 de Rijk, M. G., van Eekelen, A. P. J., Boesveldt, S., Kaldenberg, E., Holwerda, T., Lansink, C. J. M., Feskens, E. J. M., & de Vries, J. H. M. (2023). Macronutrient intake and alertness during night shifts - the time interval matters. *Frontiers in nutrition*, *10*, 1245420. https://doi.org/10.3389/fnut.2023.1245420

183 Mason, I. C., Qian, J., Adler, G. K., & Scheer, F. A. J. L. (2020). Impact of circadian disruption on glucose metabolism: implications for type 2 diabetes. *Diabetologia*, *63*(3), 462–472. https://doi.org/10.1007/s00125-019-05059-6

184 Molzof, H. E., Peterson, C. M., Thomas, S. J., Gloston, G. F., Johnson, R. L., Jr, & Gamble, K. L. (2022). Nightshift Work and Nighttime Eating Are Associated With Higher Insulin and Leptin Levels in Hospital Nurses. *Frontiers in endocrinology*, *13*, 876752. https://doi.org/10.3389/fendo.2022.876752

185 Oriyama, S., & Yamashita, K. (2021). Effects of a snack on performance and errors during a simulated 16-h night shift: A randomized, crossover-controlled, pilot study. *PloS one*, *16*(10), e0258569. https://doi.org/10.1371/journal.pone.0258569

186 Gupta, C. C., Coates, A. M., Dorrian, J., & Banks, S. (2019). The factors influencing the eating behaviour of shiftworkers: what, when, where and why. *Industrial health*, *57*(4), 419–453. https://doi.org/10.2486/indhealth.2018-0147

187 Centofanti, S., Heilbronn, L. K., Wittert, G., Dorrian, J., Coates, A. M., Kennaway, D., Gupta, C., Stepien, J. M., Catcheside, P., Yates, C., Grosser, L., Matthews, R. W., & Banks, S. (2025). Fasting as an intervention to alter the impact of simulated night-shift work on glucose metabolism in healthy adults: A cluster randomised controlled trial. *Diabetologia*, *68*, 203–216. https://doi.org/10.1007/s00125-024-06279-1

188 Gupta, C. C., Coates, A. M., Dorrian, J., & Banks, S. (2019). The factors influencing the eating behaviour of shiftworkers: what, when, where and why. *Industrial health*, *57*(4), 419–453. https://doi.org/10.2486/indhealth.2018-0147

189 Thomas, J. M., Kern, P. A., Bush, H. M., McQuerry, K. J., Black, W. S., Clasey, J. L., & Pendergast, J. S. (2020). Circadian rhythm phase shifts caused by timed exercise vary with chronotype. *JCI insight*, *5*(3), e134270. https://doi.org/10.1172/jci.insight.134270

190 Juda, M., Vetter, C., & Roenneberg, T. (2013). The Munich ChronoType Questionnaire for Shift-Workers (MCTQShift). *Journal of biological rhythms, 28*(2), 130–140. https://doi.org/10.1177/0748730412475041

191 National Heart, Lung, and Blood Institute. (2023). *Chrononutrition: Timing of meals matters for your health.* U.S. Department of Health and Human Services. https://www.nhlbi.nih.gov/news/2023/chrononutrition-timing-meals-matters-your-health

192 Mishra, S., Persons, P. A., Lorenzo, A. M., Chaliki, S. S., & Bersoux, S. (2023). Time-Restricted Eating and Its Metabolic Benefits. *Journal of clinical medicine, 12*(22), 7007. https://doi.org/10.3390/jcm12227007

193 Tricò, D., Masoni, M. C., Baldi, S., Cimbalo, N., Sacchetta, L., Scozzaro, M. T., Nesti, G., Mengozzi, A., Nesti, L., Chiriacò, M., & Natali, A. (2024). Early time-restricted carbohydrate consumption vs conventional dieting in type 2 diabetes: a randomised controlled trial. *Diabetologia, 67*(2), 263–274. https://doi.org/10.1007/s00125-023-06045-9

194 Shukla, A. P., Andono, J., Touhamy, S. H., Casper, A., Iliescu, R. G., Mauer, E., Shan Zhu, Y., Ludwig, D. S., & Aronne, L. J. (2017). Carbohydrate-last meal pattern lowers postprandial glucose and insulin excursions in type 2 diabetes. *BMJ open diabetes research & care, 5*(1), e000440. https://doi.org/10.1136/bmjdrc-2017-000440

195 Vernia, F., Di Ruscio, M., Ciccone, A., Viscido, A., Frieri, G., Stefanelli, G., & Latella, G. (2021). Sleep disorders related to nutrition and digestive diseases: a neglected clinical condition. *International journal of medical sciences, 18*(3), 593–603. https://doi.org/10.7150/ijms.45512

196 Iao, S. I., Jansen, E., Shedden, K., O'Brien, L. M., Chervin, R. D., Knutson, K. L., & Dunietz, G. L. (2022). Associations between bedtime eating or drinking, sleep duration and wake after sleep onset: findings from the American time use survey. *British Journal of Nutrition, 127*(12), 1888–1897. doi:10.1017/S0007114521003597

197 Afaghi, A., O'Connor, H., & Chow, C. M. (2007). High-glycemic-index carbohydrate meals shorten sleep onset. *The American journal of clinical nutrition, 85*(2), 426–430. https://doi.org/10.1093/ajcn/85.2.426

Exercise as the Shift Work Lifeline

198 Anderson, E., & Durstine, J. L. (2019). Physical activity, exercise, and chronic diseases: A brief review. *Sports medicine and health science, 1*(1), 3–10. https://doi.org/10.1016/j.smhs.2019.08.006

199 World Health Organization. (2024, June 26). *Nearly 1.8 billion adults at risk of disease from not doing enough physical activity.* https://www.who.int/news/item/26-06-2024-nearly-1.8-billion-adults-at-risk-of-disease-from-not-doing-enough-physical-activity

200 World Health Organization. (2025). *Physical activity.* WHO. https://www.who.int/initiatives/behealthy/physical-activity

201 Easton, D. F., Gupta, C. C., Vincent, G. E., & others. (2024). Move the night way: How can physical activity facilitate adaptation to shift work? *Communications Biology, 7,* 259. https://doi.org/10.1038/s42003-024-05962-8

202 Mamen, A., Øvstebø, R., Sirnes, P. A., Nielsen, P., & Skogstad, M. (2020). High-Intensity Training Reduces CVD Risk Factors among Rotating Shift Workers: An Eight-Week Intervention in Industry. *International journal of environmental research and public health, 17*(11), 3943. https://doi.org/10.3390/ijerph17113943

203 Hannemann, J., Laing, A., Glismann, K., Skene, D. J., Middleton, B., Staels, B., Marx, N., Grant, P. J., Federici, M., Niebauer, J., & Böger, R. (2020). Timed physical exercise does not influence circadian rhythms and glucose tolerance in rotating night shift workers: The EuRhythDia study. *Diabetes & vascular disease research, 17*(5), 1479164120950616. https://doi.org/10.1177/1479164120950616

204 Shen, B., Ma, C., Wu, G., Liu, H., Chen, L., & Yang, G. (2023). Effects of exercise on circadian rhythms in humans. *Frontiers in pharmacology, 14,* 1282357. https://doi.org/10.3389/fphar.2023.1282357

205 Sack, R. L., Brandes, R. W., Kendall, A. R., & Lewy, A. J. (2000). Entrainment of free-running circadian rhythms by melatonin in blind people. *The New England journal of medicine, 343*(15), 1070–1077. https://doi.org/10.1056/NEJM200010123431503

206 Flahr, H., Brown, W. J., & Kolbe-Alexander, T. L. (2018). A systematic review of physical activity-based interventions in shift workers. *Preventive medicine reports, 10,* 323–331. https://doi.org/10.1016/j.pmedr.2018.04.004

207 National Academies of Sciences, Engineering, and Medicine. (2021). *The future of nursing 2020–2030: Charting a path to achieve health equity* (J. L. Flaubert, S. Le Menestrel, D. R. Williams, et al., Eds.; Chapter 10, Supporting the health and professional well-being of nurses). National Academies Press. https://www.ncbi.nlm.nih.gov/books/NBK573902/

208 Alnawwar, M. A., Alraddadi, M. I., Algethmi, R. A., Salem, G. A., Salem, M. A., & Alharbi, A. A. (2023). The Effect of Physical Activity on Sleep Quality and Sleep Disorder: A Systematic Review. *Cureus, 15*(8), e43595. https://doi.org/10.7759/cureus.43595

Your HITT Rebellion

209 Mielniczek, M., & Aune, T. K. (2024). The Effect of High-Intensity Interval Training (HIIT) on Brain-Derived Neurotrophic Factor Levels (BNDF): A Systematic Review. *Brain sciences, 15*(1), 34. https://doi.org/10.3390/brainsci15010034

210 Mahatme, S., K, V., Kumar, N., Rao, V., Kovela, R. K., & Sinha, M. K. (2022). Impact of high-intensity interval training on cardio-metabolic health outcomes and mitochondrial function in older adults: a review. *Medicine and pharmacy reports, 95*(2), 115–130. https://doi.org/10.15386/mpr-2201

211 Guo, Z., Li, M., Cai, J., Gong, W., Liu, Y., & Liu, Z. (2023). Effect of High-Intensity Interval Training vs. Moderate-Intensity Continuous Training on Fat Loss and Cardiorespiratory Fitness in the Young and Middle-Aged a Systematic Review and Meta-Analysis. *International journal of environmental research and public health, 20*(6), 4741. https://doi.org/10.3390/ijerph20064741

212 Gibala, M. J., Gillen, J. B., & Percival, M. E. (2014). Physiological and health-related adaptations to low-volume interval training: influences of nutrition and sex. *Sports medicine (Auckland, N.Z.), 44 Suppl 2*(Suppl 2), S127–S137. https://doi.org/10.1007/s40279-014-0259-6

213 Kalkanis, A., Demolder, S., Papadopoulos, D., Testelmans, D., & Buyse, B. (2023). Recovery from shift work. *Frontiers in neurology, 14*, 1270043. https://doi.org/10.3389/fneur.2023.1270043

The Breakroom: Where Willpower Fades

214 Garbarino, S., Lanteri, P., Bragazzi, N. L., Magnavita, N., & Scoditti, E. (2021). Role of sleep deprivation in immune-related disease risk and outcomes. *Communications biology, 4*(1), 1304. https://doi.org/10.1038/s42003-021-02825-4

215 Lewis, R. G., Florio, E., Punzo, D., & Borrelli, E. (2021). The Brain's Reward System in Health and Disease. *Advances in experimental medicine and biology, 1344*, 57–69. https://doi.org/10.1007/978-3-030-81147-1_4

216 Daut, R. A., & Fonken, L. K. (2019). Circadian regulation of depression: A role for serotonin. *Frontiers in neuroendocrinology, 54*, 100746. https://doi.org/10.1016/j.yfrne.2019.04.003

217 Baumeister, R.F., Bratslavsky, E., Muraven, M. & Tice, D.M. (1998). Ego depletion: Is the active self a limited resource? Journal of Personality and Social Psychology, 74, 1252–1265.

218 Cheng, P., & Drake, C. L. (2018). Psychological Impact of Shift Work. *Current sleep medicine reports, 4*(2), 104–109.

219 Bhatnagar, A., Murray, G., & Ray, S. (2023). Circadian biology to advance therapeutics for mood disorders. *Trends in Pharmacological Sciences, 44*(10), 744–758. https://doi.org/10.1016/j.tips.2023.07.008

Shielding the Cell

220 Kalogerakou, T., & Antoniadou, M. (2024). The Role of Dietary Antioxidants, Food Supplements and Functional Foods for Energy Enhancement in Healthcare Professionals. *Antioxidants (Basel, Switzerland), 13*(12), 1508. https://doi.org/10.3390/antiox13121508

221 Hanna, M., Jaqua, E., Nguyen, V., & Clay, J. (2022). B Vitamins: Functions and Uses in Medicine. *The Permanente journal, 26*(2), 89–97. https://doi.org/10.7812/TPP/21.204

A Compass in the Dark

222 Masters, A., Pandi-Perumal, S. R., Seixas, A., Girardin, J. L., & McFarlane, S. I. (2014). Melatonin, the Hormone of Darkness: From Sleep Promotion to Ebola Treatment. *Brain disorders & therapy, 4*(1), 1000151. https://doi.org/10.4172/2168-975X.1000151

223   Garde, A. H., Nabe-Nielsen, K., Jensen, M. A., Kristiansen, J., Sørensen, J. K., & Hansen, Å. M. (2020). The effects of the number of consecutive night shifts on sleep duration and quality. *Scandinavian journal of work, environment & health*, 46(4), 446–453. https://doi.org/10.5271/sjweh.3885

224   James, S. M., Honn, K. A., Gaddameedhi, S., & Van Dongen, H. P. A. (2017). Shift Work: Disrupted Circadian Rhythms and Sleep-Implications for Health and Well-Being. *Current sleep medicine reports*, 3(2), 104–112. https://doi.org/10.1007/s40675-017-0071-6

225   Zanif, U., Lai, A. S., Parks, J., Roenningen, A., McLeod, C. B., Ayas, N., Wang, X., Lin, Y., Zhang, J. J., & Bhatti, P. (2025). Melatonin supplementation and oxidative DNA damage repair capacity among night shift workers: a randomised placebo-controlled trial. *Occupational and environmental medicine*, 82(1), 1–6. https://doi.org/10.1136/oemed-2024-109824

226   Garaulet, M., Qian, J., Florez, J. C., Arendt, J., Saxena, R., & Scheer, F. A. J. L. (2020). Melatonin Effects on Glucose Metabolism: Time To Unlock the Controversy. *Trends in endocrinology and metabolism: TEM*, 31(3), 192–204. https://doi.org/10.1016/j.tem.2019.11.011

227   Razavi, P., Devore, E. E., Bajaj, A., Lockley, S. W., Figueiro, M. G., Ricchiuti, V., Gauderman, W. J., Hankinson, S. E., Willett, W. C., & Schernhammer, E. S. (2019). Shift Work, Chronotype, and Melatonin Rhythm in Nurses. *Cancer epidemiology, biomarkers & prevention : a publication of the American Association for Cancer Research, cosponsored by the American Society of Preventive Oncology*, 28(7), 1177–1186. https://doi.org/10.1158/1055-9965.EPI-18-1018

228   Ferracioli-Oda, E., Qawasmi, A., & Bloch, M. H. (2013). Meta-analysis: melatonin for the treatment of primary sleep disorders. *PloS one*, 8(5), e63773. https://doi.org/10.1371/journal.pone.0063773

Small Compounds, Big Shifts

229   Ling, Z.-N., Jiang, Y.-F., Ru, J.-N., Lu, J.-H., Ding, B., & Wu, J. (2023). Amino acid metabolism in health and disease. Signal Transduction and Targeted Therapy, 8, Article 345. https://doi.org/10.1038/s41392-023-01561-z

230   Ahmadi, S., Taghizadieh, M., Mehdizadehfar, E., Hasani, A., Khalili Fard, J., Feizi, H., Hamishehkar, H., Ansarin, M., Yekani, M., & Memar, M. Y. (2024). Gut microbiota in neurological diseases: Melatonin plays an important regulatory role. *Biomedicine & Pharmacotherapy, 171,* 116487. https://doi.org/10.1016/j.biopha.2024.116487

231   Wong, S. D., Wright, K. P., Jr, Spencer, R. L., Vetter, C., Hicks, L. M., Jenni, O. G., & LeBourgeois, M. K. (2022). Development of the circadian system in early life: maternal and environmental factors. *Journal of physiological anthropology, 41*(1), 22. https://doi.org/10.1186/s40101-022-00294-0

232   Lindseth, G., Helland, B., & Caspers, J. (2021). The impact of tryptophan supplementation on sleep quality: A systematic review, meta-analysis, and meta-regression. *Nutrition Reviews, 80*(2), 361–374. https://doi.org/10.1093/nutrit/nuab027

233   Yasuo, S., Iwamoto, A., Lee, S.-i., & Ochiai, S. (2017). L-serine enhances light-induced circadian phase resetting in mice and humans. *The Journal of Nutrition, 147*(12), 2347–2353. https://doi.org/10.3945/jn.117.255380

234   Natural Health Research. (2014, August 12). *L-ornithine shown to improve stress levels and sleep quality.* https://www.naturalhealthresearch.org/l-ornithine-shown-to-improve-stress-levels-and-sleep-quality/

235   Kawai, N., Sakai, N., Okuro, M., Karakawa, S., Tsuneyoshi, Y., Kawasaki, N., Takeda, T., Bannai, M., & Nishino, S. (2015). The sleep-promoting and hypothermic effects of glycine are mediated by NMDA receptors in the suprachiasmatic nucleus. *Neuropsychopharmacology : official publication of the American College of Neuropsychopharmacology, 40*(6), 1405–1416. https://doi.org/10.1038/npp.2014.326

The Sun You Can Swallow

236   Bikle, D. D. (2025, June 15). Vitamin D: Production, metabolism, and mechanism of action. In K. R. Feingold, S. F. Ahmed, B. Anawalt, et al. (Eds.), *Endotext.* MDText.com, Inc. https://www.ncbi.nlm.nih.gov/books/NBK278935/

237   Martelli, M., Salvio, G., Santarelli, L., & Bracci, M. (2022). Shift Work and Serum Vitamin D Levels: A Systematic Review and Meta-Analysis. *International journal of environmental research and public health, 19*(15), 8919. https://doi.org/10.3390/ijerph19158919

238 Sîrbe, C., Rednic, S., Grama, A., & Pop, T. L. (2022). An update on the effects of vitamin D on the immune system and autoimmune diseases. *International Journal of Molecular Sciences, 23*(17), 9784. https://doi.org/10.3390/ijms23179784

239 Ahmadieh, H., & Arabi, A. (2023). Association between vitamin D and cardiovascular health: Myth or Fact? A narrative review of the evidence. *Women's health (London, England), 19*, 17455057231158222. https://doi.org/10.1177/17455057231158222

240 Giustina, A., Bilezikian, J. P., Adler, R. A., Banfi, G., Bikle, D. D., Binkley, N. C., Bollerslev, J., Bouillon, R., Brandi, M. L., Casanueva, F. F., di Filippo, L., Donini, L. M., Ebeling, P. R., El-Hajj Fuleihan, G., Fassio, A., Frara, S., Jones, G., Marcocci, C., Martineau, A. R., ... Virtanen, J. K. (2024). Consensus statement on vitamin D status assessment and supplementation: Whys, whens, and hows. *Endocrine Reviews, 45*(5), 625–654. https://doi.org/10.1210/endrev/bnae009

241 Voulgaridou, G., Papadopoulou, S. K., Detopoulou, P., Tsoumana, D., Giaginis, C., Kondyli, F. S., Lymperaki, E., & Pritsa, A. (2023). Vitamin D and Calcium in Osteoporosis, and the Role of Bone Turnover Markers: A Narrative Review of Recent Data from RCTs. *Diseases (Basel, Switzerland), 11*(1), 29. https://doi.org/10.3390/diseases11010029

242 Pei, Y. Y., Zhang, Y., Peng, X. C., Liu, Z. R., Xu, P., & Fang, F. (2022). Association of Vitamin D Supplementation with Cardiovascular Events: A Systematic Review and Meta-Analysis. *Nutrients, 14*(15), 3158. https://doi.org/10.3390/nu14153158

243 Huiberts, L. M., & Smolders, K. C. (2020). Effects of vitamin D on mood and sleep in the healthy population: Interpretations from the serotonergic pathway. *Sleep Medicine Reviews, 55*, 101379. https://doi.org/10.1016/j.smrv.2020.101379

244 de Oliveira, C., Hirani, V., & Biddulph, J. P. (2018). Associations Between Vitamin D Levels and Depressive Symptoms in Later Life: Evidence From the English Longitudinal Study of Ageing (ELSA). *The journals of gerontology. Series A, Biological sciences and medical sciences, 73*(10), 1377–1382. https://doi.org/10.1093/gerona/glx130

245 Athanassiou, L., Kostoglou-Athanassiou, I., Koutsilieris, M., & Shoenfeld, Y. (2023). Vitamin D and autoimmune rheumatic diseases. *Biomolecules, 13*(4), 709. https://doi.org/10.3390/biom13040709

246 Corsello, A., Macchi, M., D'Oria, V., Pigazzi, C., Alberti, I., Treglia, G., De Cosmi, V., Mazzocchi, A., Agostoni, C., & Milani, G. P. (2023). Effects of vitamin D supplementation in obese and overweight children and adolescents: A systematic review and meta-analysis. *Pharmacological Research*, *192*, 106793. https://doi.org/10.1016/j.phrs.2023.106793

Stability in the Storm

247 Jackson P. (2025). Omega-3 fatty acids and sleep: recent advances in understanding effects and mechanisms. *Current opinion in clinical nutrition and metabolic care*, *28*(2), 61–65. https://doi.org/10.1097/MCO.0000000000001095

248 Antao, H. S., Sacadura-Leite, E., Aguiar, P., Gois, C., Marques, J., Pombo, S., & Figueira, M. L. (2024). Association between omega-3 index and depersonalization among healthcare workers in a university hospital: A cross-sectional study. *Frontiers in Psychiatry, 15*. https://doi.org/10.3389/fpsyt.2024.1425792

249 National Institutes of Health, Office of Dietary Supplements. (2025). *Omega-3 fatty acids: Fact sheet for health professionals*. U.S. Department of Health and Human Services. https://ods.od.nih.gov/factsheets/Omega3FattyAcids-HealthProfessional/

250 Alijani, S., Hahn, A., Harris, W. S., & Schuchardt, J. P. (2025). Bioavailability of EPA and DHA in humans – A comprehensive review. *Progress in Lipid Research, 97*, 101318. https://doi.org/10.1016/j.plipres.2024.101318

251 Wen, J., Satyanarayanan, S. K., Li, A., Yan, L., Zhao, Z., Yuan, Q., Su, K.-P., & Su, H. (2023). Unraveling the impact of omega-3 polyunsaturated fatty acids on blood-brain barrier (BBB) integrity and glymphatic function. *Brain, Behavior, and Immunity, 115*, 341–350. https://doi.org/10.1016/j.bbi.2023.10.018

The Silent Architect

252 Fatima, G., Dzupina, A., B Alhmadi, H., Magomedova, A., Siddiqui, Z., Mehdi, A., & Hadi, N. (2024). Magnesium Matters: A Comprehensive Review of Its Vital Role in Health and Diseases. *Cureus, 16*(10), e71392. https://doi.org/10.7759/cureus.71392

253 Arab, A., Rafie, N., Amani, R., & Shirani, F. (2023). The Role of Magnesium in Sleep Health: a Systematic Review of Available Literature. *Biological trace element research*, *201*(1), 121–128. https://doi.org/10.1007/s12011-022-03162-1

254 Rawji, A., Peltier, M. R., Mourtzanakis, K., Awan, S., Rana, J., Pothen, N. J., & Afzal, S. (2024). Examining the Effects of Supplemental Magnesium on Self-Reported Anxiety and Sleep Quality: A Systematic Review. *Cureus*, *16*(4), e59317. https://doi.org/10.7759/cureus.59317

255 Nielsen, F. H. (2013). Relation between magnesium deficiency and sleep disorders and associated pathological changes. In V. R. Preedy (Ed.), *Handbook of nutrition, diet, and sleep* (pp. 401–410). Academic Press. https://doi.org/10.1016/B978-0-12-420168-2.00031-4

256 Rawji, A., Peltier, M. R., Mourtzanakis, K., Awan, S., Rana, J., Pothen, N. J., & Afzal, S. (2024). Examining the Effects of Supplemental Magnesium on Self-Reported Anxiety and Sleep Quality: A Systematic Review. *Cureus*, *16*(4), e59317. https://doi.org/10.7759/cureus.59317

257 Zhang, C., Hu, Q., Li, S., Dai, F., Qian, W., Hewlings, S., Yan, T., & Wang, Y. (2022). A Magtein®, Magnesium L-Threonate, -Based Formula Improves Brain Cognitive Functions in Healthy Chinese Adults. *Nutrients*, *14*(24), 5235. https://doi.org/10.3390/nu14245235

258 Noah, L., Dye, L., Bois De Fer, B., Mazur, A., Pickering, G., & Pouteau, E. (2021). Effect of magnesium and vitamin B6 supplementation on mental health and quality of life in stressed healthy adults: Post-hoc analysis of a randomised controlled trial. *Stress and health : journal of the International Society for the Investigation of Stress*, *37*(5), 1000–1009. https://doi.org/10.1002/smi.3051

259 Blancquaert, L., Vervaet, C., & Derave, W. (2019). Predicting and Testing Bioavailability of Magnesium Supplements. *Nutrients*, *11*(7), 1663. https://doi.org/10.3390/nu11071663

Resetting The Clock: Tools That Don't Come in a Bottle

260 Paruthi, S., Brooks, L. J., D'Ambrosio, C., Hall, W. A., Kotagal, S., Lloyd, R. M., Malow, B. A., Maski, K., & others. (2016). Consensus statement of the American Academy of Sleep Medicine on the recommended amount of sleep for healthy children: Methodology and discussion. *Journal of Clinical Sleep Medicine, 12*(11), 1549–1561. https://doi.org/10.5664/jcsm.6288

261   Ruggiero, J. S., & Redeker, N. S. (2014). Effects of napping on sleepiness and sleep-related performance deficits in night-shift workers: a systematic review. *Biological research for nursing, 16*(2), 134–142. https://doi.org/10.1177/1099800413476571

262   Blume, C., Garbazza, C., & Spitschan, M. (2019). Effects of light on human circadian rhythms, sleep and mood. *Somnologie : Schlafforschung und Schlafmedizin = Somnology : sleep research and sleep medicine, 23*(3), 147–156. https://doi.org/10.1007/s11818-019-00215-x

263   Garbarino, S., Mascialino, B., Penco, M. A., Squarcia, S., De Carli, F., Nobili, L., Beelke, M., Cuomo, G., & Ferrillo, F. (2004). Professional shift-work drivers who adopt prophylactic naps can reduce the risk of car accidents during night work. *Sleep, 27*(7), 1295–1302. https://doi.org/10.1093/sleep/27.7.1295

The Caffeine Trap

264   Pegado, E., Rodrigues, C., Raposo, H., & Fernandes, A. I. (2022). The uses of coffee in highly demanding work contexts: Managing rhythms, sleep, and performance. *Social Sciences, 11*(8), 365. https://doi.org/10.3390/socsci11080365

265   Rogers, E. J., Trotter, M. G., Johnson, D., Desbrow, B., & King, N. (2024). Caffeine improves the shooting performance and reaction time of first-person shooter esports players: A dose-response study. *Frontiers in Sports and Active Living, 6*, Article 1437700. https://doi.org/10.3389/fspor.2024.1437700

266   Gardiner, C., Weakley, J., Burke, L. M., Roach, G. D., Sargent, C., Maniar, N., Townshend, A., & Halson, S. L. (2023). The effect of caffeine on subsequent sleep: A systematic review and meta-analysis. *Sleep Medicine Reviews, 71*, 101764. https://doi.org/10.1016/j.smrv.2023.101764

267   Lieberman, H. R., Agarwal, S., Caldwell, J. A., & Fulgoni, V. L., III. (2020). Demographics, sleep, and daily patterns of caffeine intake of shift workers in a nationally representative sample of the US adult population. *Sleep, 43*(3), zsz240. https://doi.org/10.1093/sleep/zsz240

268   Drake, C., Roehrs, T., Shambroom, J., & Roth, T. (2013). Caffeine effects on sleep taken 0, 3, or 6 hours before going to bed. *Journal of clinical sleep medicine : JCSM : official publication of the American Academy of Sleep Medicine*, *9*(11), 1195–1200. https://doi.org/10.5664/jcsm.3170

Timing Coffee for Longevity and Resilience

269   Kobylińska Z, Biesiadecki M, Kuna E, Galiniak S, Mołoń M. Coffee as a Source of Antioxidants and an Elixir of Youth. Antioxidants (Basel). 2025 Feb 27;14(3):285. doi: 10.3390/antiox14030285. PMID: 40227264; PMCID: PMC11939571.

270   Wang, X., Ma, H., Sun, Q., Li, J., Heianza, Y., Van Dam, R. M., Hu, F. B., Rimm, E., Manson, J. E., & Qi, L. (2025). Coffee drinking timing and mortality in US adults. *European Heart Journal, 46*(8), 749–759. https://doi.org/10.1093/eurheartj/ehae871

271   U.S. Department of Health and Human Services, & U.S. Department of Agriculture. (2015). *2015–2020 dietary guidelines for Americans* (8th ed.). https://odphp.health.gov/sites/default/files/2019-09/2015-2020_ Dietary_Guidelines.pdf

272   Torres-Collado, L., Compañ-Gabucio, L. M., González-Palacios, S., Notario-Barandiaran, L., Oncina-Cánovas, A., Vioque, J., & García-de la Hera, M. (2021). Coffee Consumption and All-Cause, Cardiovascular, and Cancer Mortality in an Adult Mediterranean Population. *Nutrients, 13*(4), 1241. https://doi.org/10.3390/ nu13041241

Calm without Compromise

273   Dasdelen, M. F., Er, S., Kaplan, B., Celik, S., Beker, M. C., Orhan, C., Tuzcu, M., Sahin, N., Mamedova, H., Sylla, S., Komorowski, J., Ojalvo, S. P., Sahin, K., & Kilic, E. (2022). A Novel Theanine Complex, Mg-L-Theanine Improves Sleep Quality *via* Regulating Brain Electrochemical Activity. *Frontiers in nutrition*, *9*, 874254. https://doi.org/10.3389/ fnut.2022.874254

274   Baba, Y., Inagaki, S., Nakagawa, S., Kaneko, T., Kobayashi, M., & Takihara, T. (2021). Effects of l-Theanine on Cognitive Function in Middle-Aged and Older Subjects: A Randomized Placebo-Controlled Study. *Journal of medicinal food*, *24*(4), 333–341. https://doi. org/10.1089/jmf.2020.4803

275 Jie, F., Yin, G., Yang, W., Yang, M., Gao, S., Lv, J., & Li, B. (2018). Stress in Regulation of GABA Amygdala System and Relevance to Neuropsychiatric Diseases. *Frontiers in neuroscience, 12*, 562. https://doi.org/10.3389/fnins.2018.00562

276 Hidese, S., Ogawa, S., Ota, M., Ishida, I., Yasukawa, Z., Ozeki, M., & Kunugi, H. (2019). Effects of L-Theanine Administration on Stress-Related Symptoms and Cognitive Functions in Healthy Adults: A Randomized Controlled Trial. *Nutrients, 11*(10), 2362. https://doi.org/10.3390/nu11102362

277 Lundquist, C. A., Ramos, L. J., Ahmed, H., Zhang, S., & Chokroverty, S. (2023). *Sleep medicine knowledge, attitudes, and practices among medical students and primary care physicians: A global survey.* medRxiv. https://doi.org/10.1101/2023.10.01.23296182

278 U.S. Food and Drug Administration. (2007, February 5). *GRAS Notice No. 209: L-theanine.* U.S. Department of Health and Human Services. https://www.hfpappexternal.fda.gov/scripts/fdcc/index.cfm?set=GRASNotices&id=209

Fuel Without Force

279 Ferreira, G. C., & McKenna, M. C. (2017). L-Carnitine and Acetyl-L-carnitine Roles and Neuroprotection in Developing Brain. *Neurochemical research, 42*(6), 1661–1675. https://doi.org/10.1007/s11064-017-2288-7

280 Shibasaki, M., Ishikawa, K., Yamada, M., & Ichikawa, T. (2006). Effects of terguride, ropinirole, and acetyl-L-carnitine on methamphetamine withdrawal in the rat. *Pharmacology Biochemistry and Behavior, 83*(3), 403–409. https://doi.org/10.1016/j.pbb.2006.02.023

281 Freo, U., Brugnatelli, V., Turco, F., & Zanette, G. (2021). Analgesic and antidepressant effects of the clinical glutamate modulators acetyl-L-carnitine and ketamine. *Frontiers in Neuroscience, 15*, 584649. https://doi.org/10.3389/fnins.2021.584649

282 Avila, A., Lewandowski, A. S., Li, Y., & Zhang, S. L. (2025). A carnitine transporter at the blood–brain barrier modulates sleep via glial lipid metabolism in *Drosophila. Proceedings of the National Academy of Sciences, 122*(4), e2421178122. https://doi.org/10.1073/pnas.2421178122

283 Cherix, A., Larrieu, T., Grosse, J., Rodrigues, J., McEwen, B., Nasca, C., Gruetter, R., & Sandi, C. (2020). Metabolic signature in nucleus accumbens for anti-depressant-like effects of acetyl-L-carnitine. *eLife, 9,* e50631. https://doi.org/10.7554/eLife.50631

Fueling The Fatigued Brain

284 Escalante, G., Gonzalez, A. M., St Mart, D., Torres, M., Echols, J., Islas, M., & Schoenfeld, B. J. (2022). Analysis of the efficacy, safety, and cost of alternative forms of creatine available for purchase on Amazon.com: Are label claims supported by science? *Heliyon, 8*(11), e12113. https://doi.org/10.1016/j.heliyon.2022.e12113

285 Kreider, R. B., & Stout, J. R. (2021). Creatine in Health and Disease. *Nutrients, 13*(2), 447. https://doi.org/10.3390/nu13020447

286 Forbes, S. C., Cordingley, D. M., Cornish, S. M., Gualano, B., Roschel, H., Ostojic, S. M., Rawson, E. S., Roy, B. D., Prokopidis, K., Giannos, P., & Candow, D. G. (2022). Effects of Creatine Supplementation on Brain Function and Health. *Nutrients, 14*(5), 921. https://doi.org/10.3390/nu14050921

287 Chang, H., & Leem, Y. H. (2023). The potential role of creatine supplementation in neurodegenerative diseases. *Physical activity and nutrition, 27*(4), 48–54. https://doi.org/10.20463/pan.2023.0037

288 Gordji-Nejad, A., Matusch, A., Kleedörfer, S., Patel, H. J., Drzezga, A., Elmenhorst, D., Binkofski, F., & Bauer, A. (2024). Single dose creatine improves cognitive performance and induces changes in cerebral high energy phosphates during sleep deprivation. *Scientific Reports, 14,* Article 4937. https://doi.org/10.1038/s41598-024-50588-2

289 Antonio, J., Candow, D. G., Forbes, S. C., Gualano, B., Jagim, A. R., Kreider, R. B., Rawson, E. S., Smith-Ryan, A. E., VanDusseldorp, T. A., Willoughby, D. S., & Ziegenfuss, T. N. (2021). Common questions and misconceptions about creatine supplementation: what does the scientific evidence really show?. *Journal of the International Society of Sports Nutrition, 18*(1), 13. https://doi.org/10.1186/s12970-021-00412-w

290 Kreider, R. B., Jäger, R., & Purpura, M. (2022). Bioavailability, Efficacy, Safety, and Regulatory Status of Creatine and Related Compounds: A Critical Review. *Nutrients, 14*(5), 1035. https://doi.org/10.3390/nu14051035

The Mitochondrial Recalibrator

291 Yan, T., Nisar, M. F., Hu, X., Chang, J., Wang, Y., Wu, Y., Liu, Z., Cai, Y., Jia, J., Xiao, Y., & Wan, C. (2024). Pyrroloquinoline Quinone (PQQ): Its impact on human health and potential benefits: PQQ: Human health impacts and benefits. *Current research in food science, 9*, 100889. https://doi.org/10.1016/j.crfs.2024.100889

292 Yan, T., Nisar, M. F., Hu, X., Chang, J., Wang, Y., Wu, Y., Liu, Z., Cai, Y., Jia, J., Xiao, Y., & Wan, C. (2024). Pyrroloquinoline Quinone (PQQ): Its impact on human health and potential benefits: PQQ: Human health impacts and benefits. *Current research in food science, 9*, 100889. https://doi.org/10.1016/j.crfs.2024.100889

293 Shiojima, Y., Takahashi, M., Takahashi, R., Moriyama, H., Bagchi, D., Bagchi, M., & Akanuma, M. (2022). Effect of Dietary Pyrroloquinoline Quinone Disodium Salt on Cognitive Function in Healthy Volunteers: A Randomized, Double-Blind, Placebo-Controlled, Parallel-Group Study. *Journal of the American Nutrition Association, 41*(8), 796–809. https://doi.org/10.1080/07315724.2021.1962770

294 Gao, Y., Kamogashira, T., Fujimoto, C., Iwasaki, S., & Yamasoba, T. (2022). Pyrroloquinoline quinone (PQQ) protects mitochondrial function of HEI-OC1 cells under premature senescence. *npj aging, 8*(1), 3. https://doi.org/10.1038/s41514-022-00083-0

Repair from the Inside Out

295 Tenório, M. C. D. S., Graciliano, N. G., Moura, F. A., Oliveira, A. C. M., & Goulart, M. O. F. (2021). *N*-Acetylcysteine (NAC): Impacts on Human Health. *Antioxidants (Basel, Switzerland), 10*(6), 967. https://doi.org/10.3390/antiox10060967

296 Chakraborty, S., Rao, B. S. S., & Tripathi, S. J. (2025). The neuroprotective effects of N-acetylcysteine in psychiatric and neurodegenerative disorders: From modulation of glutamatergic transmission to restoration of synaptic plasticity. *Neuropharmacology, 278*, 110527. https://doi.org/10.1016/j.neuropharm.2025.110527

297 Sedlak, T. W., Paul, B. D., Parker, G. M., Hester, L. D., Snowman, A. M., Taniguchi, Y., Kamiya, A., Snyder, S. H., & Sawa, A. (2019). The glutathione cycle shapes synaptic glutamate activity. *Proceedings of the National Academy of Sciences of the United States of America, 116*(7), 2701–2706. https://doi.org/10.1073/pnas.1817885116

298 Bushana, P. N., Schmidt, M. A., Chang, K. M., Vuong, T., Sorg, B. A., & Wisor, J. P. (2023). Effect of N-Acetylcysteine on Sleep: Impacts of Sex and Time of Day. *Antioxidants (Basel, Switzerland)*, *12*(5), 1124. https://doi.org/10.3390/antiox12051124

299 Khan, S. A., Campbell, A. M., Lu, Y., An, L., Alpert, J. S., & Chen, Q. M. (2021). N-Acetylcysteine for Cardiac Protection During Coronary Artery Reperfusion: A Systematic Review and Meta-Analysis of Randomized Controlled Trials. *Frontiers in cardiovascular medicine*, *8*, 752939. https://doi.org/10.3389/fcvm.2021.752939

300 Shukla, D., Goel, A., Mandal, P. K., Joon, S., Punjabi, K., Arora, Y., Kumar, R., Mehta, V. S., Singh, P., Maroon, J. C., Bansal, R., Sandal, K., Roy, R. G., Samkaria, A., Sharma, S., Sandhilya, S., Gaur, S., Parvathi, S., & Joshi, M. (2023). Glutathione Depletion and Concomitant Elevation of Susceptibility in Patients with Parkinson's Disease: State-of-the-Art MR Spectroscopy and Neuropsychological Study. *ACS chemical neuroscience*, *14*(24), 4383–4394. https://doi.org/10.1021/acschemneuro.3c00717

301 Chakraborty, S., Rao, B. S. S., & Tripathi, S. J. (2025). The neuroprotective effects of N-acetylcysteine in psychiatric and neurodegenerative disorders: From modulation of glutamatergic transmission to restoration of synaptic plasticity. *Neuropharmacology*, *240*, 110527. https://doi.org/10.1016/j.neuropharm.2025.110527

302 Bushana, P. N., Schmidt, M. A., Chang, K. M., Vuong, T., Sorg, B. A., & Wisor, J. P. (2023). Effect of N-Acetylcysteine on Sleep: Impacts of Sex and Time of Day. *Antioxidants (Basel, Switzerland)*, *12*(5), 1124. https://doi.org/10.3390/antiox12051124

303 **The Neural Stabilizer**

Ma, X., Li, X., Wang, W., Zhang, M., Yang, B., & Miao, Z. (2022). Phosphatidylserine, inflammation, and central nervous system diseases. *Frontiers in aging neuroscience*, *14*, 975176. https://doi.org/10.3389/fnagi.2022.975176

304 Komori T. (2015). The Effects of Phosphatidylserine and Omega-3 Fatty Acid-Containing Supplement on Late Life Depression. *Mental illness*, *7*(1), 5647. https://doi.org/10.4081/mi.2015.5647

305   Valadas, J. S., Esposito, G., Vandekerkhove, D., Miskiewicz, K., Deaulmerie, L., Raitano, S., Seibler, P., Klein, C., & Verstreken, P. (2018). ER lipid defects in neuropeptidergic neurons impair sleep patterns in Parkinson's disease. *Neuron, 98*(6), 1155–1169.e6. https://doi.org/10.1016/j.neuron.2018.05.022

306   Vakhapova, V., Cohen, T., Richter, Y., Herzog, Y., & Korczyn, A. D. (2010). Phosphatidylserine containing omega-3 fatty acids may improve memory abilities in non-demented elderly with memory complaints: a double-blind placebo-controlled trial. *Dementia and geriatric cognitive disorders, 29*(5), 467–474. https://doi.org/10.1159/000310330

307   Kato-Kataoka, A., Sakai, M., Ebina, R., Nonaka, C., Asano, T., & Miyamori, T. (2010). Soybean-derived phosphatidylserine improves memory function of the elderly Japanese subjects with memory complaints. *Journal of clinical biochemistry and nutrition, 47*(3), 246–255. https://doi.org/10.3164/jcbn.10-62

308   Richter, Y., Herzog, Y., Lifshitz, Y., Hayun, R., & Zchut, S. (2013). The effect of soybean-derived phosphatidylserine on cognitive performance in elderly with subjective memory complaints: a pilot study. *Clinical interventions in aging, 8,* 557–563. https://doi.org/10.2147/CIA.S40348

Fueling The Fatigued Cell

309   Mantle, D., Hargreaves, I. P., Domingo, J. C., & Castro-Marrero, J. (2024). Mitochondrial Dysfunction and Coenzyme Q10 Supplementation in Post-Viral Fatigue Syndrome: An Overview. *International journal of molecular sciences, 25*(1), 574. https://doi.org/10.3390/ijms25010574

310   Sood, B., Patel, P., & Keenaghan, M. (2024, January 30). Coenzyme Q10. In *StatPearls*. StatPearls Publishing. https://www.ncbi.nlm.nih.gov/books/NBK531491/

311   Mousavi, S., Mohammadi, V., & Foroughi, Z. (2019). Effect of coenzyme Q10 supplementation on work-related fatigue in nurses: A double-blind, randomized placebo-controlled study. *Fatigue: Biomedicine, Health & Behavior, 8*(8), 1–10. https://doi.org/10.1080/21641846.2019.1704374

The Resilience Root

312   Ivanova Stojcheva, E., & Quintela, J. C. (2022). The Effectiveness of *Rhodiola rosea* L. Preparations in Alleviating Various Aspects of Life-Stress Symptoms and Stress-Induced Conditions-Encouraging Clinical Evidence. *Molecules (Basel, Switzerland), 27*(12), 3902. https://doi.org/10.3390/molecules27123902

313   Panossian, A., & Wikman, G. (2010). Effects of Adaptogens on the Central Nervous System and the Molecular Mechanisms Associated with Their Stress-Protective Activity. *Pharmaceuticals (Basel, Switzerland), 3*(1), 188–224. https://doi.org/10.3390/ph3010188

314   Darbinyan, V., Kteyan, A., Panossian, A., Gabrielian, E., Wikman, G., & Wagner, H. (2000). *Rhodiola rosea* in stress-induced fatigue — A double-blind cross-over study of a standardized extract SHR-5 with a repeated low-dose regimen on the mental performance of healthy physicians during night duty. *Phytomedicine, 7*(5), 365–371. https://doi.org/10.1016/S0944-7113(00)80055-0

315   Punja, S., Shamseer, L., Olson, K., & Vohra, S. (2014). Rhodiola rosea for mental and physical fatigue in nursing students: a randomized controlled trial. *PloS one, 9*(9), e108416. https://doi.org/10.1371/journal.pone.0108416

316   Chen, Y., Tang, M., Yuan, S., Fu, S., Li, Y., Li, Y., Wang, Q., Cao, Y., Liu, L., & Zhang, Q. (2022). Rhodiola rosea: A Therapeutic Candidate on Cardiovascular Diseases. *Oxidative medicine and cellular longevity, 2022*, 1348795. https://doi.org/10.1155/2022/1348795

317   Ivanova Stojcheva, E., & Quintela, J. C. (2022). The Effectiveness of *Rhodiola rosea* L. Preparations in Alleviating Various Aspects of Life-Stress Symptoms and Stress-Induced Conditions-Encouraging Clinical Evidence. *Molecules (Basel, Switzerland), 27*(12), 3902. https://doi.org/10.3390/molecules27123902

318   Tinsley, G. M., Jagim, A. R., Potter, G. D. M., Garner, D., & Galpin, A. J. (2024). *Rhodiola rosea* as an adaptogen to enhance exercise performance: a review of the literature. *The British journal of nutrition, 131*(3), 461–473. https://doi.org/10.1017/S0007114523001988

The Root That Adapts and Endures

319   National Institutes of Health, Office of Dietary Supplements. (2025, February 14). *Ashwagandha: Fact sheet for health professionals.* U.S. Department of Health and Human Services. https://ods.od.nih.gov/factsheets/Ashwagandha-HealthProfessional/

320   Lopresti, A. L., Drummond, P. D., & Smith, S. J. (2019). A Randomized, Double-Blind, Placebo-Controlled, Crossover Study Examining the Hormonal and Vitality Effects of Ashwagandha (Withania somnifera) in Aging, Overweight Males. *American journal of men's health, 13*(2), 1557988319835985. https://doi.org/10.1177/1557988319835985

321   Begemann, K., Rawashdeh, O., Olejniczak, I., Pilorz, V., Monteiro de Assis, L. V., Osorio-Mendoza, J., & Oster, H. (2025). Endocrine regulation of circadian rhythms. *npj Biological Timing and Sleep, 2,* 10. https://doi.org/10.1038/s44323-025-00010-7

322   Vaidya, V. G., Gothwad, A., Ganu, G., Girme, A., Modi, S. J., & Hingorani, L. (2024). Clinical safety and tolerability evaluation of Withania somnifera (L.) Dunal (Ashwagandha) root extract in healthy human volunteers. *Journal of Ayurveda and integrative medicine, 15*(1), 100859. https://doi.org/10.1016/j.jaim.2023.100859

REM Without Rest

323   Hutchison, I. C., & Rathore, S. (2015). The role of REM sleep theta activity in emotional memory. *Frontiers in psychology, 6,* 1439. https://doi.org/10.3389/fpsyg.2015.01439

324   Javaid, S., Farooq, T., Rehman, Z., Afzal, A., Ashraf, W., Rasool, M. F., Alqahtani, F., Alsanea, S., Alasmari, F., Alanazi, M. M., Alharbi, M., & Imran, I. (2021). Dynamics of choline-containing phospholipids in traumatic brain injury and associated comorbidities. *International Journal of Molecular Sciences, 22*(21), 11313. https://doi.org/10.3390/ijms222111313

325   Cakir, A., Ocalan, B., Koc, C., Suyen, G. G., Cansev, M., & Kahveci, N. (2020). Effects of CDP-choline administration on learning and memory in REM sleep-deprived rats. *Physiology & behavior, 213,* 112703. https://doi.org/10.1016/j.physbeh.2019.112703

326 Derbyshire, E., & Obeid, R. (2020). Choline, Neurological Development and Brain Function: A Systematic Review Focusing on the First 1000 Days. *Nutrients*, *12*(6), 1731. https://doi.org/10.3390/nu12061731

327 Gámiz, F., & Gallo, M. (2021). A Systematic Review of the Dietary Choline Impact on Cognition from a Psychobiological Approach: Insights from Animal Studies. *Nutrients*, *13*(6), 1966. https://doi.org/10.3390/nu13061966

328 Kansakar, U., Trimarco, V., Mone, P., Varzideh, F., Lombardi, A., & Santulli, G. (2023). Choline supplements: An update. *Frontiers in endocrinology*, *14*, 1148166. https://doi.org/10.3389/fendo.2023.1148166

The Plant That Restores Pattern

329 Kramer, D. J., & Johnson, A. A. (2024). Apigenin: a natural molecule at the intersection of sleep and aging. *Frontiers in nutrition*, *11*, 1359176. https://doi.org/10.3389/fnut.2024.1359176

330 Javadi, B., & Sobhani, Z. (2024). Role of apigenin in targeting metabolic syndrome: A systematic review. *Iranian journal of basic medical sciences*, *27*(5), 524–534. https://doi.org/10.22038/IJBMS.2024.71539.15558

331 Saadatmand, S., Zohroudi, F., & Tangestani, H. (2024). The Effect of Oral Chamomile on Anxiety: A Systematic Review of Clinical Trials. *Clinical nutrition research*, *13*(2), 139–147. https://doi.org/10.7762/cnr.2024.13.2.139

Sleep, Repair, and the Brain That Never Clocks Out

332 Docherty, S., Doughty, F. L., & Smith, E. F. (2023). The Acute and Chronic Effects of Lion's Mane Mushroom Supplementation on Cognitive Function, Stress and Mood in Young Adults: A Double-Blind, Parallel Groups, Pilot Study. *Nutrients*, *15*(22), 4842. https://doi.org/10.3390/nu15224842

333 Szućko-Kociuba, I., Trzeciak-Ryczek, A., Kupnicka, P., & Chlubek, D. (2023). Neurotrophic and Neuroprotective Effects of *Hericium erinaceus*. *International journal of molecular sciences*, *24*(21), 15960. https://doi.org/10.3390/ijms242115960

334 Okamura, H., Anno, N., Tsuda, A., Inokuchi, T., Uchimura, N., & Inanaga, K. (2015). The effects of *Hericium erinaceus* (Amyloban® 3399) on sleep quality and subjective well-being among female undergraduate students: A pilot study. *Progress in Molecular Biology and Translational Science, 1,* Article 006. https://doi.org/10.1016/j.pmu.2015.03.006

335 Li, C.-H., Wang, H.-C., Chen, W.-T., Hsieh, M.-T., & Wu, C.-R. (2021). *Hericium erinaceus* mycelium ameliorates anxiety induced by continuous sleep disturbance in vivo. *BMC Complementary Medicine and Therapies, 21*(1), Article 342. https://doi.org/10.1186/s12906-021-03463-3

336 Spangenberg, E. T., Moneypenny, A., Bozzo, G. G., & Perreault, M. L. (2025). Unveiling the role of erinacines in the neuroprotective effects of *Hericium erinaceus*: a systematic review in preclinical models. *Frontiers in pharmacology, 16,* 1582081. https://doi.org/10.3389/fphar.2025.1582081

337 Docherty, S., Doughty, F. L., & Smith, E. F. (2023). The Acute and Chronic Effects of Lion's Mane Mushroom Supplementation on Cognitive Function, Stress and Mood in Young Adults: A Double-Blind, Parallel Groups, Pilot Study. *Nutrients, 15*(22), 4842. https://doi.org/10.3390/nu15224842

338 Vigna, L., Morelli, F., Agnelli, G. M., Napolitano, F., Ratto, D., Occhinegro, A., Di Iorio, C., Savino, E., Girometta, C., Brandalise, F., & Rossi, P. (2019). *Hericium erinaceus* Improves Mood and Sleep Disorders in Patients Affected by Overweight or Obesity: Could Circulating Pro-BDNF and BDNF Be Potential Biomarkers?. *Evidence-based complementary and alternative medicine : eCAM, 2019,* 7861297. https://doi.org/10.1155/2019/7861297

Sleep, Mood, and the Shifted Brain

339 Guardado Yordi, E., Pérez Martínez, A., Radice, M., Scalvenzi, L., Abreu-Naranjo, R., Uriarte, E., Santana, L., & Matos, M. J. (2024). Seaweeds as Source of Bioactive Pigments with Neuroprotective and/or Anti-Neurodegenerative Activities: Astaxanthin and Fucoxanthin. *Marine drugs, 22*(7), 327. https://doi.org/10.3390/md22070327

340   Adıgüzel, E., & Ülger, T. G. (2024). A marine-derived antioxidant astaxanthin as a potential neuroprotective and neurotherapeutic agent: A review of its efficacy on neurodegenerative conditions. *European Journal of Pharmacology, 959*, 176706. https://doi.org/10.1016/j.ejphar.2024.176706

341   Abbaszadeh, F., Jorjani, M., Joghataei, M. T., Raminfard, S., & Mehrabi, S. (2023). Astaxanthin ameliorates spinal cord edema and astrocyte activation via suppression of HMGB1/TLR4/NF-κB signaling pathway in a rat model of spinal cord injury. *Naunyn-Schmiedeberg's archives of pharmacology, 396*(11), 3075–3086. https://doi.org/10.1007/s00210-023-02512-7

342   Saito, H., Cherasse, Y., Suzuki, R., Mitarai, M., Ueda, F., & Urade, Y. (2017). Zinc-rich oysters as well as zinc-yeast- and astaxanthin-enriched food improved sleep efficiency and sleep onset in a randomized controlled trial of healthy individuals. *Molecular nutrition & food research, 61*(5), 10.1002/mnfr.201600882. https://doi.org/10.1002/mnfr.201600882

343   Abdol Wahab, N. R., Meor Mohd Affandi, M. M. R., Fakurazi, S., Alias, E., & Hassan, H. (2022). Nanocarrier System: State-of-the-Art in Oral Delivery of Astaxanthin. *Antioxidants (Basel, Switzerland), 11*(9), 1676. https://doi.org/10.3390/antiox11091676

Clarity Before Sleep

344   Clayton, P., Hill, M., Bogoda, N., Subah, S., & Venkatesh, R. (2021). Palmitoylethanolamide: A Natural Compound for Health Management. *International journal of molecular sciences, 22*(10), 5305. https://doi.org/10.3390/ijms22105305

345   Rao, A., Ebelt, P., Mallard, A., & Briskey, D. (2021). Palmitoylethanolamide for sleep disturbance. A double-blind, randomised, placebo-controlled interventional study. *Sleep science and practice, 5*(1), 12. https://doi.org/10.1186/s41606-021-00065-3

346   D'Angelo, M., & Steardo, L., Jr (2024). Cannabinoids and Sleep: Exploring Biological Mechanisms and Therapeutic Potentials. *International journal of molecular sciences, 25*(7), 3603. https://doi.org/10.3390/ijms25073603

347   Inácio de Sá, M. C., & Castor, M. G. M. (2023). Therapeutic use of palmitoylethanolamide as an anti-inflammatory and immunomodulator. *Future Pharmacology*, *3*(4), 951–977. https://doi.org/10.3390/futurepharmacol3040058

Resetting the Clock from Within

348   Yasuo, S., Iwamoto, A., Lee, S. I., Ochiai, S., Hitachi, R., Shibata, S., Uotsu, N., Tarumizu, C., Matsuoka, S., Furuse, M., & Higuchi, S. (2017). L-Serine Enhances Light-Induced Circadian Phase Resetting in Mice and Humans. *The Journal of nutrition*, *147*(12), 2347–2355. https://doi.org/10.3945/jn.117.255380

349   Ohashi, M., Lee, S. I., Eto, T., Uotsu, N., Tarumizu, C., Matsuoka, S., Yasuo, S., & Higuchi, S. (2022). Intake of L-serine before bedtime prevents the delay of the circadian phase in real life. *Journal of physiological anthropology*, *41*(1), 31. https://doi.org/10.1186/s40101-022-00306-z

350   Yasuo, S., Iwamoto, A., Lee, S. I., Ochiai, S., Hitachi, R., Shibata, S., Uotsu, N., Tarumizu, C., Matsuoka, S., Furuse, M., & Higuchi, S. (2017). L-Serine Enhances Light-Induced Circadian Phase Resetting in Mice and Humans. *The Journal of nutrition*, *147*(12), 2347–2355. https://doi.org/10.3945/jn.117.255380

351   Ito, Y., Takahashi, S., Shen, M., Yamaguchi, K., & Satoh, M. (2014). Effects of L-serine ingestion on human sleep. *SpringerPlus*, *3*, 456. https://doi.org/10.1186/2193-1801-3-456

352   Rajkowska, G., & Stockmeier, C. A. (2013). Astrocyte pathology in major depressive disorder: insights from human postmortem brain tissue. *Current drug targets*, *14*(11), 1225–1236. https://doi.org/10.2174/13894501113149990156

Subtle Stimulation Behind the Scenes

353   Mitchell, E., Slettenaar, M., Meer, N. V., Transler, C., Jans, L., Quadt, F., & Berry, M. (2011). Differential contributions of theobromine and caffeine on mood, psychomotor performance and blood pressure. *Physiology & Behavior*, *104*(5), 816–822. https://doi.org/10.1016/j.physbeh.2011.07.027

354 Baggott, M. J., Childs, E., Hart, A. B., de Bruin, E., Palmer, A. A., Wilkinson, J. E., & de Wit, H. (2013). Psychopharmacology of theobromine in healthy volunteers. *Psychopharmacology, 228*(1), 109–118. https://doi.org/10.1007/s00213-013-3021-0

355 Erblang, M., Drogou, C., Gomez-Merino, D., Metlaine, A., Boland, A., Deleuze, J. F., Thomas, C., Sauvet, F., & Chennaoui, M. (2019). The Impact of Genetic Variations in ADORA2A in the Association between Caffeine Consumption and Sleep. *Genes, 10*(12), 1021. https://doi.org/10.3390/genes10121021

356 Temple, J. L., Bernard, C., Lipshultz, S. E., Czachor, J. D., Westphal, J. A., & Mestre, M. A. (2017). The Safety of Ingested Caffeine: A Comprehensive Review. *Frontiers in psychiatry, 8*, 80. https://doi.org/10.3389/fpsyt.2017.00080

A Pharmacologic Nudge

357 Schwartz J. R. (2009). Modafinil in the treatment of excessive sleepiness. *Drug design, development and therapy, 2*, 71–85. https://doi.org/10.2147/dddt.s2377

358 Czeisler, C. A., Walsh, J. K., Roth, T., Hughes, R. J., Wright, K. P., Kingsbury, L., Arora, S., Schwartz, J. R., Niebler, G. E., Dinges, D. F., & U.S. Modafinil in Shift Work Sleep Disorder Study Group (2005). Modafinil for excessive sleepiness associated with shift-work sleep disorder. *The New England journal of medicine, 353*(5), 476–486. https://doi.org/10.1056/NEJMoa041292

359 Schwartz J. R. (2009). Modafinil in the treatment of excessive sleepiness. *Drug design, development and therapy, 2*, 71–85. https://doi.org/10.2147/dddt.s2377

360 Erman, M. K., Rosenberg, R., & The U.S. Modafinil Shift Work Sleep Disorder Study Group (2007). Modafinil for excessive sleepiness associated with chronic shift work sleep disorder: effects on patient functioning and health-related quality of life. *Primary care companion to the Journal of clinical psychiatry, 9*(3), 188–194. https://doi.org/10.4088/pcc.v09n0304

Performance Without Alignment

361 Sarfraz, N., Okuampa, D., Hansen, H., Alvarez, M., Cornett, E. M., Kakazu, J., Kaye, A. M., & Kaye, A. D. (2022). pitolisant, a novel histamine-3 receptor competitive antagonist, and inverse agonist, in the treatment of excessive daytime sleepiness in adult patients with narcolepsy. *Health psychology research*, *10*(3), 34222. https://doi.org/10.52965/001c.34222

362 Guevarra, J. T., Hiensch, R., Varga, A. W., & Rapoport, D. M. (2020). Pitolisant to Treat Excessive Daytime Sleepiness and Cataplexy in Adults with Narcolepsy: Rationale and Clinical Utility. *Nature and science of sleep*, *12*, 709–719. https://doi.org/10.2147/NSS.S264140

363 Watson, N. F., Davis, C. W., Zarycranski, D., Vaughn, B., Dayno, J. M., Dauvilliers, Y., & Schwartz, J. C. (2021). Time to Onset of Response to Pitolisant for the Treatment of Excessive Daytime Sleepiness and Cataplexy in Patients With Narcolepsy: An Analysis of Randomized, Placebo-Controlled Trials. *CNS drugs*, *35*(12), 1303–1315. https://doi.org/10.1007/s40263-021-00866-1

Pharmacological Tension

364 Rosenberg, R., & Bogan, R. (2010). Armodafinil in the treatment of excessive sleepiness. *Nature and science of sleep*, *2*, 95–105. https://doi.org/10.2147/nss.s6728

365 Czeisler, C. A., Walsh, J. K., Wesnes, K. A., Arora, S., & Roth, T. (2009). Armodafinil for treatment of excessive sleepiness associated with shift work disorder: a randomized controlled study. *Mayo Clinic proceedings*, *84*(11), 958–972. https://doi.org/10.1016/S0025-6196(11)60666-6

Wakefulness When Nature Fails

366 Fuller, M. C., Carlson, S., Pysick, H., Berry, V., Tondryk, A., Swartz, H., Cornett, E. M., Kaye, A. M., Viswanath, O., Urits, I., & Kaye, A. D. (2024). A Comprehensive Review of Solriamfetol to Treat Excessive Daytime Sleepiness. *Psychopharmacology bulletin*, *54*(1), 65–86.

367 Wickwire, E. M., Geiger-Brown, J., Scharf, S. M., & Drake, C. L. (2017). Shift Work and Shift Work Sleep Disorder: Clinical and Organizational Perspectives. *Chest*, *151*(5), 1156–1172. https://doi.org/10.1016/j.chest.2016.12.007

368 Schweitzer, P. K., Rosenberg, R., Zammit, G. K., Gotfried, M., Chen, D., Carter, L. P., Wang, H., Lu, Y., Black, J., Malhotra, A., Strohl, K. P., & TONES 3 Study Investigators (2019). Solriamfetol for Excessive Sleepiness in Obstructive Sleep Apnea (TONES 3). A Randomized Controlled Trial. *American journal of respiratory and critical care medicine*, *199*(11), 1421–1431. https://doi.org/10.1164/rccm.201806-1100OC

369 Fuller, M. C., Carlson, S., Pysick, H., Berry, V., Tondryk, A., Swartz, H., Cornett, E. M., Kaye, A. M., Viswanath, O., Urits, I., & Kaye, A. D. (2024). A Comprehensive Review of Solriamfetol to Treat Excessive Daytime Sleepiness. *Psychopharmacology bulletin*, *54*(1), 65–86.

370 Rosenberg, R., Baladi, M., & Bron, M. (2021). Clinically relevant effects of solriamfetol on excessive daytime sleepiness: a posthoc analysis of the magnitude of change in clinical trials in adults with narcolepsy or obstructive sleep apnea. *Journal of clinical sleep medicine : JCSM : official publication of the American Academy of Sleep Medicine*, *17*(4), 711–717. https://doi.org/10.5664/jcsm.9006

371 Pharmaceutical Technology. (2024). *Solriamfetol hydrochloride by Axsome Therapeutics for shift work sleep disorder: Likelihood of approval.* https://www.pharmaceutical-technology.com/data-insights/solriamfetol-hydrochloride-axsome-therapeutics-shift-work-sleep-disorder-likelihood-of-approval/

Strategies Without Stimulants

372 Corkum, P., Begum, E. A., Rusak, B., Rajda, M., Shea, S., MacPherson, M., Williams, T., Spurr, K., & Davidson, F. (2020). The Effects of Extended-Release Stimulant Medication on Sleep in Children with ADHD. *Journal of the Canadian Academy of Child and Adolescent Psychiatry = Journal de l'Academie canadienne de psychiatrie de l'enfant et de l'adolescent*, *29*(1), 33–43.

373 Antle, M. C., van Diepen, H. C., Deboer, T., Pedram, P., Pereira, R. R., & Meijer, J. H. (2012). Methylphenidate modifies the motion of the circadian clock. *Neuropsychopharmacology, 37*(11), 2446–2455. https://doi.org/10.1038/npp.2012.107

374 Schwartz JR, Roth T. Shift work sleep disorder: burden of illness and approaches to management. Drugs. 2006;66(18):2357-70. doi: 10.2165/00003495-200666180-00007. PMID: 17181377.

375 News-Medical. (2023). *Stimulants and sleep.* https://www.news-medical.net/health/Stimulants-and-Sleep.aspx

Vaccine Response in Shift Workers

376 Kim, S. H., & Chae, C. H. (2024). Potential Association between Shift Work and Serologic Response to Hepatitis B Vaccination among Manufacturing Workers in Republic of Korea. *Vaccines, 12*(9), 1041. https://doi.org/10.3390/vaccines12091041

377 Garbarino, S., Lanteri, P., Bragazzi, N. L., Magnavita, N., & Scoditti, E. (2021). Role of sleep deprivation in immune-related disease risk and outcomes. *Communications biology, 4*(1), 1304. https://doi.org/10.1038/s42003-021-02825-4

378 Ruiz, F. S., Rosa, D. S., Zimberg, I. Z., dos Santos Quaresma, M. V. L., Nunes, J. O. F., Apostolico, J. S., Weckx, L. Y., Souza, A. R., Narciso, F. V., Fernandes-Junior, S. A., Gonçalves, B., Folkard, S., Bittencourt, L., Tufik, S., & de Mello, M. T. (2020). Night shift work and immune response to the meningococcal conjugate vaccine in healthy workers: A proof of concept study. *Sleep Medicine, 75*, 263–275. https://doi.org/10.1016/j.sleep.2020.05.032

379 Kohl, I. S., Garcez, A., da Silva, J. C., de Arruda, H. C., Canuto, R., Paniz, V. M. V., & Olinto, M. T. A. (2025). Association between shift work and vitamin D levels in Brazilian female workers. *Nutrients, 17*(7), 1201. https://doi.org/10.3390/nu17071201

Metrics as a Flashlight, Not a Searchlight

380 Damoun, N., Amekran, Y., Taiek, N., & Hangouche, A. J. E. (2024). Heart rate variability measurement and influencing factors: Towards the standardization of methodology. *Global cardiology science & practice, 2024*(4), e202435. https://doi.org/10.21542/gcsp.2024.35

381 Chiang L. K. (2018). Overnight pulse oximetry for obstructive sleep apnea screening among patients with snoring in primary care setting: Clinical case report. *Journal of family medicine and primary care*, *7*(5), 1086–1089. https://doi.org/10.4103/jfmpc.jfmpc_142_18

382 Nicolò, A., Massaroni, C., Schena, E., & Sacchetti, M. (2020). The Importance of Respiratory Rate Monitoring: From Healthcare to Sport and Exercise. *Sensors (Basel, Switzerland)*, *20*(21), 6396. https://doi.org/10.3390/s20216396

383 Jafleh, E. A., Alnaqbi, F. A., Almaeeni, H. A., Faqeeh, S., Alzaabi, M. A., & Al Zaman, K. (2024). The Role of Wearable Devices in Chronic Disease Monitoring and Patient Care: A Comprehensive Review. *Cureus*, *16*(9), e68921. https://doi.org/10.7759/cureus.68921

384 Baron, K. G., Abbott, S., Jao, N., Manalo, N., & Mullen, R. (2017). Orthosomnia: Are some patients taking the quantified self too far? *Journal of Clinical Sleep Medicine*, *13*(2), 351–354. https://doi.org/10.5664/jcsm.6472

385 The American Journal of Managed Care. (2023, October 9). *Wearable devices heighten symptom monitoring, health care visits for atrial fibrillation.* https://www.ajmc.com/view/wearable-devices-heighten-symptom-monitoring-health-care-visits-for-atrial-fibrillation

Neuroprotective Gold

386 Kehtari, T., Tovar, D. C., Epstein, D., & Junquera, P. (2025). From Mood to Memory: Unlocking Saffron's Potential in Brain Health. *Cureus*, *17*(4), e82924. https://doi.org/10.7759/cureus.82924

387 Cerdá-Bernad, D., Costa, L., Serra, A. T., Bronze, M. R., Valero-Cases, E., Pérez-Llamas, F., Candela, M. E., Arnao, M. B., Barberán, F. T., Villalba, R. G., García-Conesa, M. T., & Frutos, M. J. (2022). Saffron against Neuro-Cognitive Disorders: An Overview of Its Main Bioactive Compounds, Their Metabolic Fate and Potential Mechanisms of Neurological Protection. *Nutrients*, *14*(24), 5368. https://doi.org/10.3390/nu14245368

388 He, F., Chen, C., Wang, Y., Wang, S., Lyu, S., Jiao, J., Huang, G., & Yang, J. (2023). Safranal acts as a neurorestorative agent in rats with cerebral ischemic stroke via upregulating SIRT1. *Experimental and therapeutic medicine, 27*(2), 71. https://doi.org/10.3892/etm.2023.12358

389 Chauhan, S., Tiwari, A., Verma, A., Padhan, P. K., Verma, S., & Gupta, P. C. (2024). Exploring the Potential of Saffron as a Therapeutic Agent in Depression Treatment: A Comparative Review. *The Yale journal of biology and medicine, 97*(3), 365–381. https://doi.org/10.59249/XURF4540

Reading the Signals

390 Kaur, J., Khare, S., Sizar, O., & Mesfin, F. B. (2025). *Vitamin D deficiency*. In StatPearls. StatPearls Publishing. https://www.ncbi.nlm.nih.gov/books/NBK532266/

391 Martelli, M., Salvio, G., Santarelli, L., & Bracci, M. (2022). Shift Work and Serum Vitamin D Levels: A Systematic Review and Meta-Analysis. *International journal of environmental research and public health, 19*(15), 8919. https://doi.org/10.3390/ijerph19158919

392 Marden, J. R., Mayeda, E. R., Tchetgen Tchetgen, E. J., Kawachi, I., & Glymour, M. M. (2017). High Hemoglobin A1c and Diabetes Predict Memory Decline in the Health and Retirement Study. *Alzheimer disease and associated disorders, 31*(1), 48–54. https://doi.org/10.1097/WAD.0000000000000182

393 Mouliou D. S. (2023). C-Reactive Protein: Pathophysiology, Diagnosis, False Test Results and a Novel Diagnostic Algorithm for Clinicians. *Diseases (Basel, Switzerland), 11*(4), 132. https://doi.org/10.3390/diseases11040132

394 Armstrong, M., Asuka, E., & Fingeret, A. (2023, March 13). *Physiology, thyroid function*. In StatPearls. StatPearls Publishing. https://www.ncbi.nlm.nih.gov/books/NBK537039/

395 Arosio, P., Cairo, G., & Bou-Abdallah, F. (2024). A Brief History of Ferritin, an Ancient and Versatile Protein. *International journal of molecular sciences, 26*(1), 206. https://doi.org/10.3390/ijms26010206

396 Thorarinsdottir, E. H., Arnardottir, E. S., Benediktsdottir, B., Janson, C., Olafsson, I., Pack, A. I., Gislason, T., & Keenan, B. T. (2018). Serum ferritin and obstructive sleep apnea-epidemiological study. *Sleep & breathing = Schlaf & Atmung, 22*(3), 663–672. https://doi.org/10.1007/s11325-017-1598-y

397 Ankar, A., & Kumar, A. (2024, September 10). *Vitamin B12 deficiency.* In StatPearls. StatPearls Publishing. https://www.ncbi.nlm.nih.gov/books/NBK441923/

www.ingramcontent.com/pod-product-compliance
Lightning Source LLC
Chambersburg PA
CBHW052119270326
41930CB00012B/2683